WHAT IF
GLUTEN-FREE
IS **NOT** ENOUGH?

The Balance Diet - **Weight-Loss**
Connection

A 60-Day Program
By Chen Ben -Asher

Win Your Health with THE BALANCED DIET

WHAT IF **GLUTEN-FREE** IS **NOT** ENOUGH?

The **Weight-Loss** Connection

TABLE OF CONTENTS

ABOUT THE AUTHOR

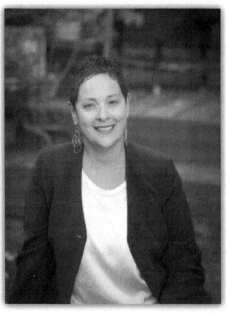

CHEN BEN ASHER IS Board Certified in Holistic Nutrition® Consultant, M.A, CGP, FLT. Chen specializes in women's health, Metabolic Syndrome, diabetes, hormonal imbalances, and weight management. She is a public speaker, educator, clinician, author, and creator of "What if Gluten Free is Not Enough?, The Weight Loss Connection", "Best Foods to Eat After Surgery", How To Reduce High URIC ACID, Candida – Functional Nutritional Approach; Step by Step – How to take control of Candida" and more.

Chen provides holistic nutritional approaches by looking for the underlying causes of your body's systems imbalances. She has worked one-on-one with hundreds of clients in person and via Skype or video in her own private Functional Nutrition practice in the Bay Area, California. Her effective "Gain Health

Lose Weight" program is a customized nutritional plan that leads to optimal wellness. The program is created to assist individuals in developing a personal strategy to support and balance their health, focusing on engagement, disease prevention, chronic and/ or acute condition management through nutrition, real foods and healthy weight maintenance.

Chen is a member of "The National Association of Nutrition Professionals" (NANP) as well as "The Holistic Nutrition Credentialing Board" (HNCB).

ACKNOWLEDGEMENT

NOBODY HAS BEEN MORE important to me in the pursuit of this project than my loving family. Above all I want to thank my husband, Mor, and our children Evyatar and Eliya, who supported, encouraged and loved me despite all the time it took me away from them in last 3 years of writing this book. I also thank my parents who raised me and inspired me to keep up with my mission in life, to bring the truth, while supporting so many individuals out there who are struggling to lose weight.

Thanks for all of those who have touched my life while losing weight, getting balanced and healthier. The tears, the laughter and joy we shared as part of the nutritional and lifestyle changes that we all went through together while shaping the content of this book.

Thanks for my two great editiors, Bonnie Jo Davis and Gabriel Reynolds who both skillfully, patiently and brilliantly brought this master piece to completion.

To all who provided support, read, wrote, offered comments, allowed me to quote their remarks and assisted in the editing, proofreading and design.

And to my friends that where patiently waiting until I reached the finish line, thank you.

INTRODUCTION

Before diving into the details of this book, I would like to take a moment to share my story with you, primarily because you probably have a similar story that you could share with me about your own life. The first memory I have of struggling to lose weight was when I was 15 years old. I was on a field trip with my class when a classmate made an obnoxious comment. Little did I know at the time that this incident would be a life-changing moment. As you probably know, at about 15 you begin to notice that the opposite gender is paying more attention to your looks. Of course, this also leads to learning how to do your eyelashes and flirt a little too!

It was a hot summer day, and I was in my cute little shorts. I was passing by a group of giggling girls when I overheard one of them saying: *"Look at her! She's so fat!"* My face turned bright red as I walked away feeling downcast.

Hearing what that girl said made me feel like someone slapped me. I was never petite, but I didn't ever think I was fat. Her comment changed how I viewed myself and it was a starting point for my long struggle with weight cautiousness.

Struggling to lose weight is an experience many of us have in common. We are all very familiar with the hunger that comes from following a strict diet and the frustration it brings. We follow or have tried a million different diets. We have practiced willpower and have often bravely said "no" when offered a dessert. We get frustrated when the number on the bathroom scale does not change. We often suffer from health issues since we follow diets that do not necessarily fit our bodies' needs. Just like many others, I also struggled to lose weight for many years. Hence, it is very important to note that I have been down this exact same path!

When I look back at pictures of myself, I see that I wasn't actually fat when I was 15. I was young, balanced, and happy (5'7", 125 lbs.). However, I was somehow brainwashed into feeling uncomfortable about how I looked.

I cut calories and started to work out. I tried many different diets: low carb, low sugar, vegetarian, and more. Just name it, and I've probably tried it! I never followed a single diet that did not make me feel hungry. I lost weight only to gain it back and then lose it again. Sound familiar?

My moods changed and my monthly period was inconsistent when I was stressed, tired, or frustrated. I constantly battled my weight. The drag on my academics was almost inevitable.

Over the years, every crisis in my life, big or small, led to another cycle of gaining weight, adding to my stress and frustration. Unfortunately, I later discovered I had intestinal yeast overgrowth, which is called "gut dysbiosis." Besides my energy drain, I had constant diarrhea, headaches, and difficulty breathing. I was a busy mother, wife, and worker. I pushed myself to a point where I had to figure out what was wrong.

That is when I decided to change my diet. I took a food allergy test and discovered I'm allergic to gluten, dairy, eggs, some nuts and seeds, and, most surprisingly, olive oil! Regardless of the nutritional benefits olive oil has for others, my body does not get along with it. In fact, when I consume olive oil, it creates a negative hemoglobin reaction in my body – a reaction with multiple adverse effects if not taken good care off. This means, in spite of the fact that I was eating healthy food, it wasn't necessarily good for my body. As soon as I discovered my body's intolerances and allergies, I started taking care of myself and became my own nutritionist. It took me ten months to get completely off gluten. It was a gradual process which required a lot of learning and practice. I even learned that I was required to eat more quantities of certain foods to maintain and balance my weight. Subsequently, I stopped eating foods I was sensitive or allergic to.

My constant struggle with my weight was a professional journey that lead me to see weight as a representation of health and balance rather than a measure of beauty. I realized that I needed to nourish my body to feel balanced, empowered, and energetic. I learned how to eat the right foods in the right quantities. This is how my body could maintain the healthy balance that it needed without getting to a point where I was hungry and ill.

The right method for many of my clients and myself is maintaining a balanced lifestyle with the right nutritional plan.

There's an old saying that knowledge is power. There's no doubt that having knowledge about which foods are beneficial to you is incredibly important for maintaining a healthy lifestyle. It is so powerful that you can control, reverse, or prevent many chronic conditions and illnesses just by understanding which foods your body can handle! For example, even though olive oil is known for having extraordinary nutritional benefits, I know now I cannot consume it because I'm allergic to it.

When I entered the nutritional field, it became clear to me that I needed to share this mindset with others. The Balance Diet is not the classic model of starvation nor over-working yourself in the gym or God forbidden, taking "magic" diet pills, it is all about, **nourishing your body and maintaining balance in a natural way.**

The quality of the food is more important than the quantity. This doesn't necessarily mean it's important to eat organic versus GMO (Genetically Modified Organism) foods, but it does mean you should eat foods that are suitable for your body's functionality.

I take a holistic approach to maintaining stable and healthy weight, in addition to reading the useful blood markers of my clients. This means I use a blend of science and technology with the healing powers nature has already provided us with.

My all-inclusive holistic practice is based on nutritional and lifestyle changes. Over time, I have developed methods, customized nutrition plans, explored lifestyle changes and constructed a support system which motivated me to write this book about the balanced diet. This balanced diet has already proven to be successful in helping most of my clients realize there is no such thing as a universal diet that works for everybody. Once a person acknowledges this fact, they can reduce their weight and maintain it for more than 12 months, just by harnessing the power of understanding what is happening inside their bodies!

No person should have to keep struggling with their weight! It doesn't matter if they are children, teens or adults. They all deserve to feel good about themselves! Nobody should have to go through the crazy roller-coaster of diets, mood swings, and disease. By adapting your diet and eating properly in accordance with your body's requirements, you will nourish yourself, reduce stress, and maintain your overall well-being in the future.

THE GLUTEN-FREE WEIGHT
LOSS CONNECTION

In our hectic daily lives, we are surrounded by high-calorie foods and snacks, making it difficult to avoid or resist unhealthy eating. Not to mention that it is harder than ever to stay active! Unfortunately, this makes it incredibly easy to consume a lot more calories than our bodies need.

The first step most people take when they start any weight-loss diet is cutting down their calorie intake, which simply means they are consuming less food. They'll lose some pounds at first, but shortly after, they will regain the weight back. Studies will support my clinical observations, showing that between 80% and 95% of dieters will regain their lost weight after quitting their diet. [*2,8] Additionally, it's revealed that two thirds of individuals who re-gain weight end up even fatter after quitting the diet than they were before the diet. [*6] Even on a gluten-free diet, the results are similar. On average, people gain about 16.6 pounds after quitting a gluten free diet. In a study done over 1000 subjects over three years on a gluten free diet, 22% of the subjects gained weight. Their Body Mass Index (BMI) was increased by >2 pts, and 17% who started at a normal weight crossed over into being overweight or obese. [*4,6] Another study conducted by Dickey & Kearney in 2006 reported that after two years on a gluten free diet, 82% of their 143 overweight and obese patients with Celiac disease had gained weight. [1]   Additionally, in a study published by the European Journal of Internal Medicine in 2012, Ukkola and Mäki revealed that 69% of the underweight patients from a sample of 698 gained weight on a gluten free diet after a year. 18% of overweight patients and 42% of obese patients lost weight, though the rest of the patients' BMI remained stable. [9]

One can argue and say that it is hard to draw any conclusions out of this small number of studies and sample sizes. However, this pattern of losing some pounds at first, and regaining them back by quitting the diet, no matter if the patient is on gluten free diet or not, is similar.

Some people might wonder why someone would think cutting gluten out of their diet would help them lose weight. Well, the general assumption is that eliminating or reducing gluten from one's diet causes quick and easy weight loss.

If you choose to avoid gluten, you will most likely feel better at first. You will probably replace the gluten with more vegetables, fruits, proteins, and fats (nuts and seeds). They will provide you with plenty of nutrients, so at the beginning of the diet, you may feel better and, feel more energetic, and even lose weight! However, this incredible experience is not permanent. In most cases, the flaws of the gluten-free diet will begin to appear after a few months. Most commonly, people start to report that cutting back on gluten increases their calories intake. Also, they feel increased cravings for sweets as well as carbohydrates. This craving leads to uncontrolled munching on cheap, convenient and ready-to-go foods. Consequently, the results are obvious; regaining all the lost weight is almost inevitable!

Unless you have been diagnosed with Celiac disease or gluten sensitivity you should not follow a gluten-free diet as a weight loss program. If you are hoping to lose weight quickly or to change how you feel you are risking your health by avoiding gluten like many other millions of people who get fatter and fatter and fatter every year.

When currently overweight individuals gain weight after excluding gluten, it becomes a potential cause of morbidity. The prescribed gluten-free diet needs to be modified accordingly to better suit that specific individual's body and metabolism.

In fact, as of right now, there is not a enough published reports supporting the claim that following a gluten-free diet will lead to weight loss in people who are not suffering from Celiac disease (related to the abdomen) or gluten sensitivity. Clearly, there is no hard scientific evidence to support such a claim. In fact, a 2011 article published in the *Journal of the American Dietetic Association* states: "At this time, there is no scientific evidence supporting the alleged benefit that a gluten-free diet will promote weight loss." [1]

OKAY, SO WHO SHOULD GO ON A GLUTEN-FREE DIET?

In my opinion, no one should eliminate gluten from their diet just for the sake of losing weight. However, some medical conditions leave people with no choice. If you do choose to go on a gluten-free diet without legitimate health reasons such as Celiac disease, food allergies or food sensitivity to grains containing gluten; you are simply rolling the dice with your health.

Many people with biopsy-diagnosed Celiac disease are malnourished, overweight, or obese before starting a gluten-free diet. [1,7] A restricted gluten-free diet does not lead to any weight loss for them at all. Unfortunately, weight gain is common [4] in overweight or obese adults as well as children with celiac disease when they go on gluten-free diets.

A 2012 study of 1,018 patients with confirmed biopsies shows people diagnosed with Celiac disease gained weight when going gluten-free. 16% of patients moved from an average or low BMI class into an overweight BMI class. 22% of the patients who were overweight at the time of diagnosis gained more weight after starting their strict gluten-free diet. [3]

There are additional side effects apart from the weight gain. In most cases, people with Celiac unfortunately they suffer diarrhea, reduced hemoglobin concentration, reduced bone mineral density, osteoporosis, and higher grades of villous atrophy which erodes away the microscopic, finger like tentacles on the small intestines. In the study, 81% of patients on a gluten-free diet had gained weight within 2 years while 82% of them started as overweight.

Individuals with Celiac disease must deal with those dietary constrictions and their consequences. Unfortunately, individuals with Celiac disease or gluten sensitivity have no choice, but if you do not have celiac disease, you do have a choice! If you have not been diagnosed with celiac disease or any condition that requires you to stop consuming gluten, and if you are not known with allergies or sensitives to gluten, then you should not go on a gluten-free diet. It's that simple!

LOSING CONTROL

BODY SIGNALS FOR NUTRIENT DEPLETION

As DISCUSSED EARLIER IN this book, the first step most people take when they start any weight loss program is cutting back on their daily calorie intake. Many people will reduce their carbohydrate, sugar and flour intake as well. The rationale of carbohydrate restriction is in response to lower glucose availability and changes in insulin and glucagon concentrations which direct the body away from fat storage moving towards fat oxidation. [*5]

To the surprise of many, cutting back on calories does not serve as an effective weight loss tool for a healthy lifestyle. Typically, the average person cuts about 20% to 40% of their total energy intake, which is an average of about 300 to 600 calories per day.

Unfortunately, when starting a diet, most individuals are already nutritionally depleted, over-stressed, and hormonally imbalanced. Cutting back on calories pushes their biological mechanisms further into the red zone by reducing the circulation of several hormone levels. Growth factors and cytokines (small proteins released by cells which alert underlying causes that may lead to anticancer effects, negative signaling pathways, inflammation as well as cellular and systemic homeostasis pathways) which does not support maintaining a healthy weight.

In fact, this leads to increased serious risks for many chronic conditions such as heart disease, diabetes, autoimmune disease, and cancer, as well as many other ailments such as sleep apnea (pauses in breathing or shallow breathing during sleep), high blood pressure, high blood sugars, joint problems, and even psychological problems. [*4]

Research shows that about 80-95% of people will regain weight around 3 to 4 months after they start a low carbohydrate diet. In most cases, they will end up heavier than they were at their starting point. [*7]

This phenomenon of regaining weight corresponds to my clinical observation: the simple model of creating a **negative energy balance** by reducing caloric consumption and/or increasing physical activity is not effective. More specifically, cutting back on calories even if you are on a low carbohydrate diet **will not do you any good!**

On a self-led weight loss dieting program, many people will cut back an average of 300 to 600 calories per day. This means their calorie intake is below the recommended daily requirement which will affect the metabolic rate (amount of energy used while resting in a neutrally temperate environment). This is how the process of regaining weight starts.

PROCESS OF REGAINING THE WEIGHT OR WEIGHT LOSS RESISTANCE

The ineffective method of cutting down calories starts a metabolic slowdown which affects the blood sugar levels and lowers energy levels. In such circumstances, bodily functions become compromised.

Signs like irritation, decreased body temperature, low energy and hunger due to a slow metabolic rate (BMR - Basal Metabolic Rate), amount of energy expended while resting in a neutrally temperate environment) will be present. The cravings for sweets, salt, fatty foods and carbohydrates will increase as the body tries to balance energy levels. [*4]

When you feel hungry, you lose control of the quality and quantity of food you consume. Keeping weight at a healthy level requires **eating whole, dense foods full of macro and micro nutrients,** which balance your well-being.

What you should be doing is nourishing your body with more calories coming from foods your body can tolerate so you can function better and prevent potential diseases while maintaining a healthy and balanced weight.

People make incorrect assumptions when they don't consume carbohydrates (one of the most important types of nutrients) as their primary energy source. They think they'll be able to shift from glucose (simple sugar) and fatty acids as a source of energy to fatty acids and ketones (chemical substances that can be indicators of further diseases). However, this only leads to a reduced appetite presenting the illusion they are achieving their primary goal of weight loss. The actual reality is ketones will be produced by our bodies to burn fat even when there is not enough glucose or fatty acid to be utilized as a source of energy. The body will also produce ketones if there's not enough insulin to metabolize sugar for energy. High levels of ketones are toxic to the body! This condition is called ketoacidosis. It is most commonly found with type 1 diabetes as well as with people with type 2 diabetes, though it's less likely. Severe cases of ketoacidosis can even be fatal! [*6]

The dangers of triggering a slow metabolic rate last longer than the period you were dieting or cutting back on food. Surprisingly, the negative effects last even if you regain your weight back creating a potentially bigger problem.

The metabolism damage can last for months and even years in extreme cases. People can develop "weight loss resistance" (a condition making it challenging and almost impossible to lose or keep weight off), chronic fatigue, immune suppression (reduced activity or efficiency of the immune system), food or environmental sensitivities, allergies, malnutrition, sleep apnea, and hormonal imbalances such as thyroid challenges, adrenal fatigue, over insulin production, sexual hormones imbalances, depression, and anxiety. These require even longer periods of time to reverse and bring into balance. [*1]

In my clinical experience, leading individuals through the BALANCE "Gain Health, Lose Weight" nutritional support system which I developed, I consistently hear these claims: "I cut back on gluten," "I'm spending hours in the gym every week," "I'm exhausted," "I only eat greens, but there's no weight change on the scale," or "How come we both eat the same foods, but I don't lose weight and he does?" I hear it over and over again! These men and women are putting so much effort into losing weight, cutting back on gluten, carbohydrates, sugars, going Paleo, juicing, fasting, or exercising without significant changes. When you have developed "weight loss resistance" it takes longer to nourish your body and balance it. Only then will you lose weight.

BODY CHALLENGES FROM A GLUTEN-FREE DIET

The gluten-free diet presents unique challenges for the body. It's far from being the optimal diet. When you cut gluten out as one of your food sources to try losing weight, one of the first natural bio-reactions is a slowed metabolism. In other words, you will feel hungry! This is the body's natural, self-protective response to cutting calories, or more specifically cutting a source of fuel. Your body recognizes the limited energy supply and will slow its metabolism to conserve energy while prolonging vital organ functionality (such as heart, brain, liver and kidney function) under these new stressful circumstances.

It's true that the body burns fat for fuel, but lean muscle mass will be used for fuel as well. As a consequence, these processes will slow down your metabolism much further, and eventually leading to fatigue, mood swings, and nutrient deficiencies. This condition affects the heart, lungs, and nervous system. It increases inflammation (body's response to irritation which causes swelling, pain, etc.), challenges your digestive system and sleep, and causes hormonal imbalances. In addition to all those health challenges, you will regain your weight, which is counterproductive to the reason for the gluten-free diet in the first place!

Think of your body as a balanced bank account. The core principle is managing a delicate balance between spending and saving. To be balanced, you need to nourish yourself with proper nutrients: clean, organic, non-GMO, dense, real food, which helps to maintain balance.

The optimum balanced bank account can be achieved by knowing your sources of income. The same holds true within our body. It's important to know your food sources as well as understand if your body recognizes that food as being beneficial (even if the food is considered to be healthy it might not react well with your body) without involving your immune system (see additional information in the food sensitivity section). You could be sensitive or allergic to certain foods, which might disrupt your body's delicate balancing system or "bank account." This leads to becoming overweight. By having access to this data, you could project your expenses and manage your body's bank account properly and effectively.

We all want to have a balanced, stable, and healthy body, similar to our bank account. We can work hard with no results or we could work smarter and achieve an optimum healthy weight.

Our daily budget planning process is divided by known and unexpected variables. Known variables such as food (groceries), utilities (monthly bills for water, electricity, gas, phone, internet, etc.), car payments, insurance, mortgage payments, insurance, taxes, etcetera) are all planned and budgeted. However, unexpected variables must be considered such as car accident repair, replacing your refrigerator, major dental treatment, or God forbid losing a job and having to rely on savings! You get the picture and the same goes for our bodies, too.

If you eat healthy food according to your body's needs, you will be rewarded with a healthy and balanced body. If not, you will get yourself into unpleasant and expensive debt in the form of potential disease. We all agree that planning a realistic budget, setting priorities, and practicing saving methods is the key towards stable financial freedom. The same holds true regarding monitoring our body's nutrient intake.

The heavy toll that our bodies pay for the decision to go on a gluten-free diet without a justified medical reason is not clear yet. Don't get me wrong, though, people who are diagnosed with gluten sensitivity or allergies must be on a gluten-free diet! **However, they need to be highly conscious of specific nutrients or supplements needed in their daily diet to keep their body balanced and less depleted.**

When hungry, you are vulnerable and more likely to consume the available food in an uncontrollable manner, regardless of its quality. We call it "comfort food," but the fact is, we crave comfort foods when our bodies require more fuel to function!

When constantly hungry, you will find yourself reaching a point of self- starvation. Furthermore, people on starvation diets are highly susceptible to inevitably regaining all weight lost as soon as they embark on a regular eating cycle. It's an inescapable circle that has already been proven. The resultant stress caused on your body is huge, and it prevents you from obtaining proper nutrients and energy. This only brings potential health challenges in the long run. Some of these health issues may include vitamin or mineral deficiency, anemia, diarrhea, rashes, edema (swelling from excess fluid in the cavities or body's tissues), hormonal imbalances such as adrenal fatigue (from a poorly working adrenal gland), hyperthyroidism or hypothyroidism (overproduction of thyroxine hormone), high cholesterol levels, vitamin D deficiency, blood serum glucose level imbalance, testosterone and estrogen level imbalance (most likely, sex hormones will decrease during starvation mode), sexual drive diminishing, gastrointestinal problems, autoimmune diseases, and in more severe cases even heart failure!

GLUTEN-FREE PRODUCTS: ARE THEY TRULY HEALTHIER?

Gluten-free foods are not necessarily healthier than gluten-full ones. The number one reason consumers choose to purchase gluten-free products is because they are perceived to be healthier than their gluten-full counterparts. [*3] If you are gluten-free because you are trying to lose weight, you will find yourself eating much more of the gluten-free replacement products, thinking they are a much healthier option for you.

Unfortunately, most gluten-free products have not been proven to be healthier. The replacement ingredients for wheat gluten are based on mixtures containing high glycemic index fibers and proteins from soy, potatoes, rice, corn, barley, and cereal binding starches. When consumed in excess, these alternatives may lead to high glucose levels, estrogen dominant hormonal balances, inflammation, weight gain, and digestive challenges like diarrhea, constipation, bloating, gas, fermentation, and intestinal overgrowth of bacteria like candida.

Gluten-free products could satiate your hunger, but you have to remember these products are high in calories, fats, saturated fats, vegetable oils, and sugar. They contain fewer beneficial nutrients such dietary fibers, vitamins, minerals, and complex carbohydrates. The logical statement we hear so often is to avoid "processed foods." Shouldn't it be the same with "processed gluten-free foods"? Unfortunately, avoiding processed food will not apply if you feel hungry or if you feel low in energy. Replacing your body's nutrient needs with no nutritional value replacements only worsens your health while negatively affecting your glucose and insulin levels. Over time, this will also cause your inflammation blood markers to change, which eventually stresses your body and stops you from losing weight. **Every bite counts, even if it's gluten-free!**

When you eliminate carbohydrates completely, you are on a Diet that is known as the Atkins Diet. However, if you are on gluten-free Diet and eat all the gluten-free grains available, you will gain weight.

Don't be fooled by marketing or advertising by the food industry or even some of the medical community members. They are trying to make you believe that gluten-free products are healthier options. Use your instincts and listen to your body's needs. Processed food is processed food, even if it's gluten free. Obviously, if you have been diagnosed with celiac (an autoimmune disease) or found gluten sensitive, you have to avoid gluten, but you shouldn't completely rely on processed gluten-free foods for nourishment.

LOW CARBOHYDRATE DIET
VS. GLUTEN-FREE DIET

W
HEN PEOPLE BEGIN A low carbohydrate diets to lose weight, they usually limit their carbohydrate intake by reducing their consumption of grains, legumes, beans, starchy vegetables and fruits. Primarily, people try this by switching to a gluten-free diet in an attempt to eliminate their carbohydrate consumption entirely.

Low carbohydrate diets and gluten-free diets are not exactly the same. However, both are very similar and have different health benefits. Despite the hundreds of studies being done regarding these two diets, the information can still be confusing. Understanding the differences between these two diets will help you make better choices to achieve improved health as well as a balanced weight.

A. LOW CARBOHYDRATE DIET - BENEFITS AND CHALLENGES

With a low carbohydrate diet, a person limits his or her intake of carbohydrates while consuming more protein and fats instead. The daily carbohydrate food intake on a low carbohydrate diet varies. The general dietary suggestion is a limit of 60 to 130 grams of carbohydrates; this provides between 300 to 600 calories a day. This is about 50% less than the Dietary Guidelines for Americans regarding the consumption of carbohydrates. The recommended number of calories per day is 2,000. From this amount, about 900 to 1,300 calories (225 to 325 grams) are carbohydrates.

The basis of a low carbohydrate diet is to control blood sugar levels. When you eat carbohydrates, blood sugar levels are elevated as they stimulate the release of insulin from the pancreas. Insulin regulates blood sugar levels by signaling for the liver, muscles, and fat cells to utilize glucose from the blood as an energy source.

Carbohydrates are stored in two different areas of the body -- the muscles and the liver -- as a new form known as glycogen. Any stored glycogen will also include 3-4 grams of water, which is reflected in your overall weight. [2]

When energy sources are available, excess glucose circulating in the body will be stored as glycogen by the liver from insulin signals. The liver can store up to 5% of its mass as glycogen and up to 40% of it its weight in fat.

In simpler terms, the more carbohydrates you eat, the more glycogen and water will be stored. Unfortunately, this results in increased weight. This is the reason why most individuals will experience fast and easy weight reduction within the first 10-20 days of cutting back on carbohydrates (gluten-free or not). You see, one pound of fat stored equals 3,500 calories! This also requires one pound of water storage.

Carbohydrates are found in grains (gluten-free or not), beans, legumes, fruits, starchy vegetables, milk, nuts, seeds, and, of course, unhealthy processed sources such as sugary cereals, crackers, cakes, flours, jams, preserves, bread products, refined potato products, and sugary drinks. Carbohydrates, sugars, and starches are broken down into monosaccharide units or simple sugars (glucose) during digestion. These are used by the body as an energy source.

There are three main types of carbohydrates in food: starches, sugars, and fibers. These serve as a source of fuel for the body.

a. Starchy foods:

Starch can be found in various types of food. It is important to know where it comes from in order to follow a low carbohydrate diet.

1. **Starchy vegetables**: Beets, cassava, daikon, parsnips, potatoes, pumpkins, rutabaga, spaghetti squash, sweet potatoes, turnips, winter squash, peas, corn, and yams

2. **Beans and legumes:** zuki, anasaki, black, black eye peas, fava, garbanzo, kidney, lima, mung, navy, pink, pinto, soy and lentils

3. **Grains:** wheat, rice, wild rice, oat, barley, spelt, kamut, farro, millet, teff, corn, amaranth, sorghum and buckwheat

b. Sugar foods:

Sugar is a natural substance that occurs in a variety of foods as well as commercially produced goods. There are several distinct types of sugars, which are classified by their chemical structure. A single sugar molecule is classified as a monosaccharide. This is the simple sugar: glucose, fructose, and galactose. Two single sugar molecules are called disaccharides; sucrose, maltose, and lactose and two single sugars bound together are called polysaccharides. One gram of sugar contains four calories. Most of us think about excess of sugar as refined sugar. However, excess of sugar can be found also in healthy foods. So, let's look at some common sugars found in foods, so you can make better choices.

1. **Dextrose** also known as **glucose**: A simple monosaccharide (sugar) and an important carbohydrate source. Glucose is one of the main products of photosynthesis and it starts cellular respiration (set of

metabolic reactions and processes within body cells) and is the primary sugar used to feed most living cells. Excess glucose in the blood may result in elevated insulin levels, which may damage insulin receptor sites and imbalance overall blood sugar levels. This raises insulin tolerance, which affects your weight.

2. **Lactose:** Disaccharide composed of glucose and galactose also known as "milk sugar." Lactose makes up 2-8% of milk. Lactose is a byproduct of the enzyme mammals produce to break lactase down.

3. **Fructose:** This simple sugar (monosaccharide) is found in many foods and is one of the three important dietary monosaccharides. Fructose combined with glucose makes sucrose (table sugar). Fructose is found in many foods, including most fruits, honey, and some vegetables such as beets, sweet potatoes, parsnips, and onions. Fructose has the sweetest taste of all the naturally occurring carbohydrates and is 1.73 times sweeter than table sugar. It is also worth knowing that excess fructose consumption may result in insulin resistance, weight gain, obesity, elevated LDL cholesterol, triglycerides (type of fat), metabolic syndrome, gout, and non-alcoholic fatty liver disease.

4. **Maltose:** Disaccharide (double sugar), also known as malt sugar, formed from two units of glucose. Maltose can be broken down by hydrolysis into two glucose molecules. Maltose is an important part of the brewing process and is often produced from germinated cereal grains such as barley. Maltose is used often in food and beverage production.

5. **Sucrose** also known as **table sugar**: Disaccharide is composed of glucose and fructose. Sucrose is the most commonly used food sweetener and is the most important sugar found in plants. It is commonly extracted

from sugar cane or beets and then purified. Sucrose can also be commercially derived from maple syrup and sorghum (a grain, forage or sugar crop). Sucrose is an easily digested and absorbed macronutrient which assimilates across digestive membranes and raises blood sugar rapidly.

6. **Added sugars:** Found in processed sweeteners such as high fructose corn syrup, rice syrup, beet sugar, table sugar, brown sugar, molasses, honey, cane sugar, confectioner's sugar, powdered sugar, raw sugar, maple syrup, agave nectar and sugar cane syrup.

c. Fiber foods:

Dietary fibers are an integral part of the plant-based foods we eat. These fibers are naturally found in the fruits, vegetables, nuts, and grains we consume. Dietary fibers are not digested by our intestines and most of them pass through. All dietary fibers are either soluble or insoluble. Both types of fiber are equally important for health and digestion, as well as the prevention of conditions such as heart disease, diabetes, obesity, diverticulitis (inflammation of a diverticulum), and constipation. Most plant foods have a mix of both fibers. According to WHO (The World Health Organization) recommendations, we need to consume 20-40 grams of dietary fibers a day, which includes both soluble and insoluble fibers. Most Americans do not consume even close to enough fiber in their diet! [5, 6]

The two main types of fibers are soluble and insoluble fibers:

1. **Soluble fibers**: Bind with fatty acids and slow digestion so blood sugars are released slower into the body. They are found in vegetable peelings as well as fruit and bran portions of whole grains. They have a beneficial effect on insulin sensitivity, which may help to control diabetes.

Soluble fibers delay the emptying of your stomach and make you feel full for longer periods. These fibers help lower LDL (bad) cholesterol and help to regulate blood sugar levels for people with diabetes. They eliminate bio-waste and, therefore, reduce weight. [*7,8,9,10]

Food sources of soluble fiber: Any of the gluten grains will provide you with soluble fibers. Gluten grains include oatmeal, oat cereal, brown rice, pasta (whole wheat, white), oat bran, beans, strawberries, nuts, flaxseeds, dried peas, blueberries, psyllium (a form of fiber), cucumbers, celery, apples, pears, oranges, passion fruit, avocado, Brussels sprouts, figs, sweet potatoes, asparagus, turnips, edamame, broccoli, apricots, nectarines, collard greens, eggplants, peaches, mangos, grapefruits, potatoes, okra (a tall-growing plant in the mallow family), beets, bananas, carrots, soy, nuts, and seeds.

2. **Insoluble fibers:** Insoluble fibers help hydrate and move waste through the intestines while controlling the pH level in the intestines. These fibers help prevent constipation and remove bio-waste faster while protecting against colon cancer.

Food sources of insoluble fiber: These are found in some vegetables and fruits as well as in legumes such as beans and peas. When water is added to food, the soluble fiber thickens and becomes sticky, gummy, and almost gel like. Soluble fiber can help slow the digestion of food. Sources of soluble fiber include whole wheat, whole grains, gluten-free grains such as teff, sorghum, rice, quinoa, millet, flax, buckwheat, amaranth, oats, wheat bran, corn bran, seeds, nuts, barley, and couscous. Bulgur can also add insoluble fibers to your diet. Other sources include vegetables such as zucchini, celery, broccoli, cabbage, onions, tomatoes, carrots, cucumbers, green beans, root vegetable skins, and dark leafy vegetables. Fruits will do the same. They result in better digestion, fewer toxins, and more weight loss!

3. **Commercial fibers:** Commercial fibers have been isolated and extracted from plant or animal sources and added to drinks and food products to boost their fiber content.

The following chart shows the most common types of dietary and functional fibers:

Types of Fiber	Soluble or Insoluble	Sources	Health Benefits
Cellulose, some hemicellulose	Insoluble	Naturally found in nuts, whole wheat, whole grains, bran, seeds and edible brown rice.	"Nature's laxative": Reduces constipation, lowers risk of diverticulitis and can help with weight loss.
Inulin oligofructose	Soluble	Extracted from onions and byproducts of sugar production from beets or chicory root. Can be added to processed foods to increase fiber.	May increase beneficial bacteria in the gut and enhance immune functionality.
Lignin	Insoluble	Found naturally in flax, rye and some vegetables.	Benefits heart health and possibly immune function. Use caution if celiac or gluten intolerant.

Mucilage, beta-glucans	Soluble	Naturally found in oats, oat bran, beans, peas, barley, flaxseed, berries, soybeans, bananas, oranges, apples and carrots.	Helps lower bad LDL cholesterol and, reduces risk of coronary heart disease and type 2 diabetes. Use caution if celiac or gluten intolerant.
Pectin and gums	Soluble (some pectins can be insoluble)	Naturally found in fruits, berries and seeds. Can also be extracted from citrus peel and other plants. Used to boost fiber in processed foods.	Slows the passage of food through the intestinal GI tract and helps lower blood cholesterol.
Polydextrose polyols	Soluble	Added to processed foods as a bulking agent and sugar substitute. Made from dextrose, sorbitol and citric acid.	Adds bulk to stools and helps prevent constipation. May cause bloating or gas.
Psyllium	Soluble	Extracted from rushed seeds or husks of the planta go ovata plant. Used in supplements and fiber drinks. Often added to foods.	Helps lower cholesterol and prevent constipation.

		Starch in plant cell walls. Naturally found in unripe bananas, oatmeal and legumes. Also, extracted and added to processed foods to increase fiber.	
Resistant starch	Soluble	Starch in plant cell walls. Naturally found in unripe bananas, oatmeal and legumes. Also, extracted and added to processed foods to increase fiber.	Helps weight management by increasing the feeling of satiety.
Wheat dextrin	Soluble	Extracted from wheat starch. Widely used to add fiber to processed foods.	Helps lower cholesterol (LDL and total cholesterol), reduces risk of coronary heart disease and type 2 diabetes. Avoid if celiac or gluten intolerant.

Source: WebMD Medical Reference [*1,3,10]

How much food fibers we need to eat?

Men and women over the age of 18 should consume at least 21-38 grams of the total dietary fiber of both kinds each day. There is need to increase ones' fiber intake to get as close as possible to 40 grams a day. If you currently do not consume enough fiber, you want to gradually increase your fiber intake to avoid stomach ache, bloating, and gas. Always drink enough water to prevent constipation. It is true that a low carb diet will cause most individuals to consume less fiber than needed.

As you can see, carbohydrates are an integral part of many food groups. When you choose to lose weight on a low carb diet, you will be able to lose pounds due to your self-restriction from a fair number of calories. However, it will be hard to maintain your new weight for a long period of time. This is often called the "yo-yo" diet phenomena. You will regain back your weight. Recent studies show no significant difference in terms of weight twelve months after starting a low carb diet compared to either a high protein or high fat diet. In fact, a year after, the difference was only about one pound, which is about 0.4 kilograms. [*4]

Low carb diets challenge our bodies. In most cases, people will be likely to experience slight headaches, bad breath, weakness, fatigue, constipation, diarrhea, vitamin and mineral deficiencies, bone loss, and increased risk of chronic diseases. This happens in the beginning of process. In extreme cases, a potential bio-mechanism called ketosis will occur. Ketosis is a condition where the body breaks down stored fats as a source of energy instead of using glucose. This increases acidity, inflammation, heart disease, and even cancer risk.

B. THE GLUTEN-FREE DIET

What is it a Gluten-free Diet?

On a gluten-free diet, a person excludes the protein gluten from his or her diet. This diet is suggested mainly for individuals that tested sensitive to gluten or have been diagnosed with Celiac disease. By eliminating gluten, a person will break the cycle of eating foods with gluten, which causes inflammation present in many systems of the body including the small intestines.

The epidemiology of gluten-related disorders has gradually risen to an estimated 5% of the global population. An estimated 1% of Americans have celiac disease, gluten sensitivity, or food allergies. Thousands of other Americans are adopting the gluten-free diet for various reasons. Some choose it to either boost their energy levels, reduce inflammation, lower glucose levels, reduce carbohydrates, or lose weight. [*8,10,27,71] However, this begs the question: is this the right decision to make or will there be later discoveries that a gluten-free diet is the wrong choice for people without gluten sensitives?

Wheat provides about 20% of the world's calories. This is the most nourishing source of food, and many people are more than determined to avoid it. The food pyramid guide recommends up to 11 servings per day of the bread, cereal, rice, and pasta group with 50% coming from whole grain sources per day. A survey conducted in 2010 at an annual celiac conference in Columbus, Ohio provided a snap-shot of alternative grain consumption among 174 conference attendees. 80% of the sampled population consumed less than half the amount of grain servings recommended by the U.S., Department of Health's Dietary Guidelines. Only 1% of the sample population consumed 6 serving a day. The results are clear: even people with no celiac are consuming less grains than they should and therefore missing the opportunity of the nutritional benefits of grains, regardless if it is gluten-free or not. [*72]

Challenges of Starting a Gluten-Free Diet

The gluten-free diet requires a great deal of time and effort in the beginning. Cutting gluten out of your diet if you've found out you're sensitive or allergic is not the only step you need to take to stay balanced and lose weight. It is a massive shift in lifestyle and food choices that requires shopping, chopping, chewing, and, of course, reading labels. You also must make sure you're **eating enough to stay satisfied.** In my case, I tested positive for gluten sensitivity, but I was not diagnosed with celiac disease. I adopted a gluten-free diet in 2005 and discovered that gluten is just one part of my food sensitivities and allergies. It took me almost ten months to completely cut gluten from my diet.

There is no easy way to adopt a gluten-free diet, but with the right attitude and knowledge, you should. The challenge is learning to **keep yourself satisfied and nourished** while replacing gluten with real food. Supporting the nutrient deficiencies with high-quality food and dietary supplements that will help you maintain balanced health and a healthy weight is paramount.

The gluten-free diet is made up of both labeled and unlabeled gluten-free foods. If a morsel of food is not labeled gluten-free, consumers must look for the ingredients **wheat, barley, rye, malt, soy, oats,** and **brewer's yeast**. If the food is a meat, poultry, or egg product, consumers also should look for the ingredients **modified food starch, dextrin,** and **starch**. It is essential that individuals receive up-to-date, timely and on-going counseling from a certified practitioner such as nutritionists proficient in Celiac disease and the gluten-free diet. This is not meant to discourage you from being gluten-free, if this is a choice you make and not a medical need. In both cases, it is helpful to work with someone who can support your health nutritionally.

As a professional nutritionist, I deal with many clients that began a gluten-free diet in hopes of losing weight. More Americans are gaining weight and becoming unhealthy by using gluten-free products that are not necessarily healthy for them. A gluten-free diet will not make you lose weight faster or at all. The gluten-free diet might deplete you off nutrients if you do not take the right steps to nourish and balance your body. [*19]

So, What is gluten?

Gluten is a class of proteins within wheat, (including spelt, semolina and durum) barley, rye and triticale (a hybrid), known collectively as prolamins. It is difficult to digest. Furthermore, gluten is composed of two different proteins called glutenin and gliadin. These two proteins were initially classified based upon their alcohol solubility, and it was thought that only gliadin triggered an immune system response. Conversely, recent studies have proven this incorrect. Glutenin can also trigger an immune system response. [*23,65]

GLUTEN TWO DIFFERENT PROTEINS

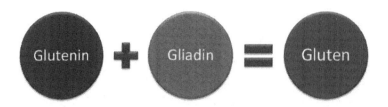

Diving deeper into the "Gluten" breakdown, it becomes even more challenging and at the same time fascinating to understand that gluten per-se might NOT be the only particle challenging your immune system and your weight. Below you will find a chart that gives you the breakdown of wheat and gluten.

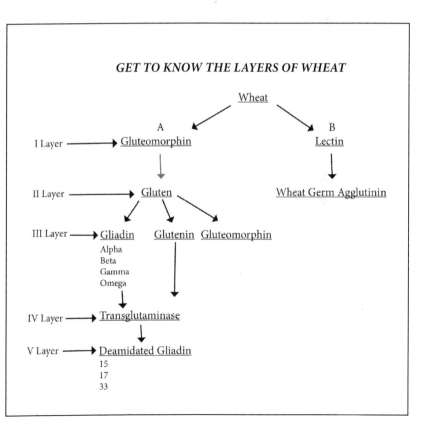

The first known layer of wheat is: **Glutemorphin and lectin.**

A. Glutemorphin breaks down to three key components which are: **gliadin, glutenin and glutemorphin:**

1. **Gliadins** - There are four different types of gliadin peptides epitopes: alpha, beta, gamma, and omega. Most labs will measure only the Alpha-Gliadin antibodies but not the Beta, Gamma, and Omega-gliadin. Unfortunately, not all people will respond to the alpha-gliadin when tested. In fact, studies show that only 50% of a sample population will respond to the alpha-gliadin test but not to the other three gliadins and glutenin epitopes. [18,40] In such cases, it may look like they are not sensitive or allergic to gliadins. They will keep eating wheat and as a result their health will be challenged and losing weight seems nearly impossible.

FOUR TYPE OF GLIADINS - THE GLUTEN PART IN WHEAT

Gliadins →	**Alpha -Gliadin**
	Beta – Gliadin → **Which One Affects You?**
	Gamma - Gliadin
	Omega – Gliadin

2. **Glutenin** – is one of the major polymeric proteins in wheat that makes 47% of the total protein content. Glutenin provides the elasticity and is rich in glycine residues in addition to other hydrophobic residues. [31,54]

3. **Gluteomorphin** is the opioid peptide that forms during digestion of the gliadin of the gluten protein. This is what makes it so difficult to remove wheat and wheat products from your diet. Some people feel terrible when they remove gluten from their diet. To make it more

challenging, the body will produce **prodynorphins.** This substance acts as an opioid and as a building block of endorphins. Endorphins are a key component in our brain. Endorphins make us feel good and happy. They improve memory and regulate perceptions of pain. People who can't produce enough prodynorphins are at risk for drug addiction, schizophrenia, bipolar disorder, and epilepsy. We know that people with gluten sensitivity can produce prodynorphins antibodies which can lead to **neurochemical disorders.** [*9,63]

THE OPIOID EFFECT OF THE BRAIN

Gluteomorphin → **Neurochemical Disorders**

A.1 Transglutaminase – is the enzyme that attaches to a protein, removes the amino groups, and replaces itself with another protein or attaches to an existing protein without the amino groups. Transglutaminase is produced to break down the gluten in wheat. It is a chemical reaction that occurs in the intestines, thyroid, heart, skin, and hair. It produces the toxin ammonia. This process is helpful in the crosslinks of the connective tissue. In individuals with gluten sensitivity, the gut will get inflamed due to the interaction between the gluten toxins and the transglutaminase enzymes. Therefore, it increases inflammation and antibody production in different sites in the body such as **Myelin Antibodies, Cerebellum Antibodies, Parietal Antibodies, Islet Cell Antibodies, Thyroid Peroxidase Antibodies, Cardiolipin Antibodies, Intrinsic Factor Antibodies and GAD 65 Antibodies.** These antibodies will lead to **autoimmune diseases** where the body attacks itself.

If you are on a gluten-free diet because you are sensitive to gluten, your health may improve dramatically because your body will **NOT** produce Transglutaminase to digest the gluten. This means less damage and less self-destruction.

TRANSGLUTAMINASE MAY LEAD TO AUTOIMMUNE DISEASES

Transglutaminase → Autoimmune Diseases

A.2 Deamidated Gliadin is another function in the process of breaking down gluten protein which will increase an immune response. While testing, we are looking for the Deamidated Gliadin 15-MER, 17-MER and 33-MER. There are two main reasons why our bodies will produce Deamidated Gliadin:

   a. A byproduct of Transglutaminase – this converts glutamines to glutamic acid and activates the immune system and tissue damage.

FIRST KNOWN REASON FOR IMMUNE RESPONSE

Gluten→ Transglutaminase → Deamidated Gliadin → Immune Response

---

   b. Deamidated Gliadin is added by the food industry to commercial and processed food since gliadins are soluble in alcohol and cannot be mixed with other foods without changing the product qualities. You want to avoid food that is labeled with wheat isolates. You can find it in food emulsifiers, starch agents, meat products, sauces, soups, salad dressing and sometimes even in red wine. [*9,24,37]

> **SECOND KNOWN REASON FOR IMMUNE RESPONSE:**
>
> **Gluten → Deamidated Gliadin → Immune Response**
>   added by the food industry
>   making the product more water soluble

B. Lectin breaks down to wheat germ agglutinin (WGA).

1. **Lectin** is part of the wheat plant defense mechanism against fungi and insects. Humans have a hard time digesting these proteins and they cause tissue damage, nutrient deficiencies, and abnormal biological reactions. Lectin is found mainly in high concentrations in whole grains, sprouted grains, and bean forms. So, if your body produces WGA antibodies, you better be off gluten.

2. **Agglutinin** (WGA) is the next step of the lectin component breakdown. It is the process that occurs when the lectins attach to the sugars or to the carbohydrates on the surface of human cells, activating pro-inflammatory chemical messengers as white blood cells. This leads to inflammatory conditions in individuals who find it difficult to digest wheat. Furthermore, agglutinin weakens the immune system, creating neurotoxins that can cross the blood-brain-barrier affecting the endocrine system. The direct tissue damage and/or the immune response does NOT require any genetic susceptibility. [14,39]

Wheat gluten is more challenging and complicated than it seems. These biological reactions can support your health, or they can cause you more harm than good. Therefore, most people find this challenging and confusing. It becomes clear that getting off gluten for the purposes of losing weight ONLY, is not entirely the right decision.

Let's Get Smart About Gluten – Prolamines, Lectins, and Phytic Acid

Most grains contain toxic proteins called **prolamines**. These proteins protect the plans. Grains such as rice, quinoa, corn and oat have prolamines as well. It is not just wheat. Prolamines are hard for humans to digest. Gliadin in wheat, Avenin in oat, Orzenin in brown rice, and Zein in corn are all prolamines that will trigger inflammatory pathways. Besides, many plants contain carbohydrates-binding proteins called **lectins** - a protein that binds reversibly to specific mono - or oligosaccharidcs. These sugar binding proteins do not digest well and trigger inflammatory pathways, an autoimmune reaction in the small intestine which leads to nutrient depletions. When we're over-consuming these grains, they bind to our metal ions while competing for the bioavailability of our self-minerals. This may lead to further nutrient depletion.

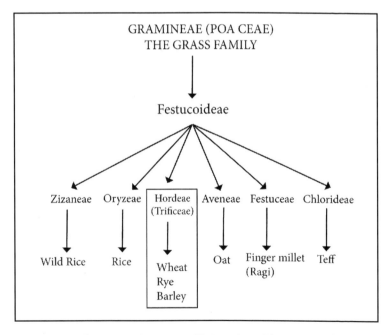

Source: United European Gastroenterol J. 2015 Apr; 3(2): 121 135
https://www.ncbi.nlm.nih.gov/pmc/articles/PMC4406897/

It can be a shock to consider that even rice contains gluten that could trigger the immune system response the same way wheat gliadin does. It may be a good starting point to avoid eating wheat. However, this does not give you the entire picture. Avoiding "trigger foods" is not the only issue you should consider. Gliadin, the gluten in wheat grain, plays a key role in promoting weight gain, insulin secretion, and inflammation. Gluten does not break down easily in the body because it is extremely hydrophobic (fail to mix with water) and contains disulfide bonds. [73]

Beans, legumes, and **nuts** contain phytic acid, which is another natural component found in plants. Phytic acid will block the absorption of iron, zinc, and calcium. [21,25,62] The challenge is how your body digests these foods and if you over-consume them, most likely your nutrient levels are low.

A PATHWAY TO A NUTRIENT DEPLETION

Grains/Beans/Nuts → inflammatory pathways → Nutrients → Disease
* Lectins   in the small intestines   depletion
* Prolamines
* Phytic acid

These groups of natural plant base toxins can lead to potential damage on the intestinal wall, leaky gut, and eventually an autoimmune reaction in addition to creating nutrient deficiencies.

Studies shows that soaking, sprouting, and fermenting these types of food will reduce levels of toxins, which will ease your ability to digest it. [1,21,61] Taking a simple action like soaking your beans prior to cooking them will help you to digest them efficiently and maintain your nutrient levels.

In the following table, you will see the percentage of total protein in each grain so you can make a better decision about which grain may be safer for your health.

Grain	Gluten (class of proteins)	% Total Protein
Wheat	Gliadin	60
Rye	Scalin	30-50
Oat	Avenin	12-16
Millet	Panicin	40
Corn	Zien	55
Rice	Orzenin	5
Barley	Hordein	46-52
Sorgum	Kafirin	52
Teff	Penniseiten	11

Are Oats and Rice Gluten-Free?

You can see from the table above that even **oats** and **rice** are not gluten-free. These grains will NOT be a safe substitute for those who experience inflammatory immune reaction, even if you don't have an immediate reaction. Over time, the damage will appear on the tissue level based on your genetic disposition. Even the **oat protein** will produce antibodies, T-cells, and IFN-y. Both represent inflammatory responses. [*8,10,27,7]

In order for food to be labeled gluten-free it must contain less than 20ppm (parts per million) of gluten, which is the size of a bread crumb. This small amount of gluten can create an immune response if you are allergic or sensitive. Oats contain 12-16% of the protein avenin. It is true that compared to wheat, it is a much lower number (60% versus 16%) and it's possible that this is the reason people react less to eating oats. Even if the package states that the food inside is gluten-free, you need to check for yourself. It is impossible to take gluten out of grains and oats completely. If consumed, it will create a chronic inflammation which is the main precursor to disease and tissue damage.

In August of 2013, the U.S. Food and Drug Administration (FDA) issued a regulation that defined the term "gluten-free" for food labeling. This food labeling regulation is critical for people with Celiac disease as foods that contain gluten trigger the production of antibodies that attack and damage the lining of the small intestine. Such damage limits the ability of Celiac disease patients to absorb nutrients with the risk of other severe health problems, including nutritional deficiencies, osteoporosis, growth retardation, infertility, miscarriages, short stature, and intestinal cancers. [*16]

Most people can tolerate gluten in small amounts. Those who have Celiac disease or gluten sensitivity might face a negative bio-reaction that may lead to health stress based on their gene expressions. It may result in the development of a gap between the cells in the small intestine, causing them to open too wide and to allow in toxins, parasites, fungi, bacteria and/or food that is not completely digested. It may also cause gluten fragments to cross the intestinal villous into the bloodstream. These substances will be recognized by the immune system as invaders or pathogens. This will activate the immune system, causing inflammation and damage to the inside of the small intestine. [*20,28,74]

What Grains and Starches Are Considered GLUTEN-FREE?

You already understand the challenges of the gluten-free diet. Luckily, markets are full of healthy, organic, dense and tasty products based on gluten-free grains and starchy vegetables that can be eaten as an alternative source to wheat or soy. I recommend eating those products, grains and starchy vegetables in **rotation and in moderation,** even if you are not found to be allergic or sensitive to gluten. If you want to lose weight, you should consume no more than ½ cup of any grain or starch vegetable, as a serving, per meal.

Here are the gluten-free grains and starches you can easily include in your diet:

Grains:

- Amaranth
- Buckwheat
- Millet
- Quinoa
- Rice, Wild Rice, Forbidden Rice
- Sorghum
- Teff

Starches:

- Arrowroot
- Beans (such as: Black, Navy, Pinto, Soy, Lentils)
- Cassava
- Peas
- Beets, Potatoes, Sweet Potatoes, Yams
- Sago
- Tapioca
- Yucca

Nuts and Seeds Flour:

- Almond Flour
- Chestnut Flour
- Coconut Flour
- Hazelnut Flour
- Flaxseed
- Chia Seeds
- Hemp Flour
- Amaranth Flour

At the same time, you want to look at the following list of **grains and starches to avoid** since they carry <u>**hidden gluten:**</u>

- Bromated Flour
- Bulgur
- Couscous
- Durum Flour
- Enriched Flour
- Emmer (Farro)
- Einkorn
- Farina
- Flour, White Flour
- Gluten Flour
- Graham Flour
- Kamut
- Kasha
- Matzo Meal/Bowl
- Phosphated Flour
- Plain Flour
- Self-rising Flour
- Semolina
- Spelt
- Triticale

Again, if you are on a gluten-free diet due to health reasons, you MUST avoid these grains and starches. If you don't have a gluten sensitivity or celiac disease, it is wise to include some of these grains in your diet, in small amounts and in rotation. Food diversity will nourish your body and keep you in balance

THE SOY BEAN CHALLENGE

Gluten Cross-Contamination Vs. Hidden Gluten

Many processed foods, including gluten-free products, contain soy. Soy is considered a "gluten-free" bean. Soy by itself is a controversial food. Soybeans are commonly grown in rotation with wheat crops, going through the same methods of harvest, same storage facilities, same transportation and thus, subject to **gluten cross-contamination,** which means: gluten-free foods that come in contact with gluten. Most restaurants cannot avoid gluten (or any food allergy) cross contamination. Many times, they will cook your gluten-free pasta in the same pot they cooked wheat pasta earlier, and unfortunately, you will have a reaction. Specify your needs if you are eating in restaurants or the homes of others so you can protect yourself from immune response and simply try to cook your own food more. **Take control of your weight and your health.**

Gluten cross contamination is NOT **hidden gluten**. Hidden gluten is a food that has gluten in it, and your immune system will respond if you are found to be allergic or sensitive. Hidden gluten can be found in other products that may surprise you.

Here is a list of products that may have gluten in them:

- Envelopes or stamps that you lick.
- Sauces for meats, hot dogs, deli meats
- Salad dressing
- Toothpaste
- Shampoo, lotions
- Makeup
- Food starches
- Food emulsifiers
- Food stabilizer
- Artificial food coloring

- Malt extract, flavor and syrup
- Dextrins
- Frying oils
- Shared cutting boards or utensils
- Grain based sweetener (i.e. malt, corn sugar)
- Thickening agents used in processed foods
- Medication (ask your pharmacists)
- Food supplements
- Seasoning
- Soy products, sauces
- Sauces, marinades, gravies
- Pet foods
- Candy
- Canned soups

As you can see, gluten is found in many products, so being on a true gluten-free diet requires adjustments that are doable, but difficult to follow. Soy is one of those hidden substance that can affect your weight if you are found to be gluten sensitive or allergic.

Is Soy A Gluten-Free Bean?

Again, pure soy beans are not a source of gluten. However, individuals with celiac disease, autoimmune disease, gluten sensitivity, gut challenges, chronic inflammation of the intestinal mucosa, or atrophy of intestinal villi may experience difficulties in digesting soy proteins. Like wheat gluten, the side effects can be nutrient malabsorption, gut bacteria, wasting, and diarrhea that leads to imbalances and weight gain. [*19,23,62,72]

Many processed foods, including gluten-free products, contain soy. It is a cheap subsidized ingredient that may affect our health and weight. You must be careful with soy intake, even if it is a plant based protein. Soy isoflavones have high levels of phytoestrogens. The three major classes of phytoestrogens are: **xenoestigens, genistein, and daidzein.** All these isoflavones have a similar structure to the human estrogen hormone, disrupting the endocrine system both in men and women, leading to weight gain. [14,25,39,65,73]

The food industry tried to remove the negative impact of including soy in so many processed foods. However, studies linked the presence of phytoestrogens to cancer cells growth, imbalance of infertility hormones - mainly progesterone and estrogen – thyroid hormone diseases and more. Soy is classified by the FDA as one of the top eight allergens and the most derived GMO (Genetically Modified Organism). [21] Other studies showed a cause active relationship between soy proteins and higher body weight and fat percentage. [1,32,64,67,76] Soy is also high in phytates. Phytates are antioxidants found in grains, beans, nuts, and seeds that bind to our bodies' minerals, mainly calcium, magnesium, zinc, iron, manganese, and potassium, which depletes our nutrient levels. [7,26,46]

Any of these negative pathways will not support your goal to lose weight. On the contrary, it is known to cause weight gain.

Soy beans are also high in calories. If you are looking to lose weight by replacing gluten with soy products, you must be aware of the calories. Herein, I gathered the best list of calories from different comprehensive nutritional resources so it will be easy to choose a soy product:

Soy Product	Serving Size	Calories
Soybean Raw	1 cup	About 775
Soy milk	1 cup	About 830
Cooked soy	1 cup	About 287
Miso	1 cup	About 547

Tempeh	1 cup	About 320
Natto	1 cup	About 371
Soy flour	1 cup	About 366
Soy Sauce (Shoyu) (Low Sodium)	1 tbsp	About 10
Soy Sauce (Tamari)	1 tbsp	About 11
Soy Sauce (Made From Hydrolyzed Vegetable Protein)	1 tbsp	About 7
Soybeans edamame (cooked)	½ cup	About 120

Suyrai, a Japanese 43-year-old female, came to my clinic to lose weight. Soy was her one food staple. In our nutritional journey, we found out that she's sensitive to soy and has a hard time digesting soy protein. Once we took soy out of her diet and replaced it with other grains and bean alternatives, she lost 15 pounds in less than 6 months. Soy was the missing link for her unexplained weight gain.

If you are sensitive or allergic to gluten, like Suyrai you want to avoid soy, even if it's organic or non-GMO. Eating soy may trigger your immune system. If you want to purchase soy products, make sure that they are certified gluten-free. This requires food manufactures to use organic raw materials and test at less than 10ppm of glutens. As mentioned before, the U.S. Food and Drug Administration's gluten-free labeling rules, specify gluten-free foods if it is less than 20 parts per millions of glutens.

I suggest you look carefully at the labels of the food you buy. There are plenty of alternatives without soy on the market. Check your dietary food supplements and medication ingredients as well. You will be surprised to find soy in so many products. Test for food sensitivity if necessary, and make a smart choice of what will be best for your body's needs.

WHY HAVE WE BECOME SO SENSITIVE TO GLUTEN?

The most dominant theory given for this massive explosion of gluten sensitivity, autoimmune diseases, inflammation, and gluten-related disorders is that most grains have been genetically modified and hybridized, so gluten content was boosted. A century ago, grain contained far less gluten, which made it chewier and more elastic than it is now.[*42]

This is only one negative impact of the **additives** and "improvers" that the food industry chooses to use within their commercial and processed foods. It increases the chance of gluten toxicity, gluten sensitivity, and even gluten allergies. We do consume far more gluten than ever before in history. Although it seems that so many of us are sensitive and allergic to gluten, it is still a small portion of the population. According to the Chicago Celiac Disease Center, an average of one out of every 133 healthy people in the US are challenged by digestive issues and diagnosed with Celiac disease.[*28,66] Also, the chemicals involved with GMO grains may explain the rise of gluten sensitivity. The first chemical is **glyphosate,** which changes, destroys, and kills healthy gut bacteria which leads to gut dysbiosis and SIBO (Small Intestinal Bacteria Overgrowth). The second chemical is **Bt-toxins** which punch holes in human cells – mainly in the gut leading to leaky gut and autoimmune disorders that, overstress and weaken our immune systems, depleting nutrients and enzymes.[*29,41,55,56]

CELIAC (GLUTEN ALLERGY) VS. WHEAT ALLERGY (WA) VS. NON-CELIAC GLUTEN SENSITIVITY (NCGS) – WHAT'S THE DIFFERENCE?

Let's clear the confusion between the terms Celiac Disease (Gluten allergy), wheat allergy (WA), and non-Celiac gluten sensitivity (NCGS). These are the medical conditions that differentiate levels of food sensitivities, specifically levels of wheat-gluten ingestion. It is important to understand the differences between the three terms, especially if you chose a gluten-free diet so you can lose weight. While on a gluten-free diet, you will improve your gastrointestinal symptoms, assuming they are an immune response to gluten. If you are not diagnosed with one of these conditions, your body will miss wheat grain as a source of energy. The term "gluten related disorders" is an umbrella name to describe all conditions related to indigestion of gluten containing food.

What is the Different?

Celiac (Gluten Allergy) is an autoimmune disease. The ingestion of gluten is genetically preconditioned in those individuals carrying the HLA (Human Leukocyte Antigen) type II DQ2 and DQ8. HLA-DQ2 and HLA-DQ8 are a group of genes that are important for the immune system. These genes may trigger the T-cell mediated immune reaction against tissue transgluaminase (tTG). This is an enzyme that leads to the intestinal mucosal damage and villous atrophy. [34,36] The autoimmune inflammatory cascade is located mainly in the small bowel. It leads to the classical enteropathy with diarrhea, weight loss, weight gain, IBS (Irritable Bowel Symptoms), Hypertransaminasemia (elevated blood liver transaminase enzymes), brain cerebellum ataxia (the cerebellum becomes inflamed or damaged), peripheral neuropathy, and malabsorption, mainly of iron, B12, and calcium syndrome. 25% of people diagnosed with celiac disease also suffer from autoimmune disease, diabetes, infertility, and thyroid diseases. Approximately 95% of patients with Celiac Disease have the HLA-DQ2 heterodimer proteins encoded by the DQA1/05 and DQB1/02 alleles. While, only 5% have the HLA-DQ8 heterodimer proteins encoded by the DQA1/03 and DQB1/0302 alleles [79, 80.] Though, we should remember, that while 30% of the population carries these two gene (HLA-DQ2 and -DQ8), only 5% of these at-risk individuals, will develop celiac disease. Factors like gastrointestinal infections, gut microbiome status, age when gluten was introduced as an infant, length of time of breast-feeding, medication usage and other genetic and environmental factors can cause Celiac disease. [*48,49] If you fall into this category, you do NOT have any choice but follow a gluten-free diet for the rest of your life.

Wheat allergy (WA) is another immunologic reaction to wheat. In this case, the Immunoglobulin E (IgE) antibodies will mediate an inflammatory response to the Monomeric Soluble Gliadins proteins: alpha-amylase, gliadins, and glutenins. [*59] It can be a life-threatening issue for some people when the IgE mediated responses could be related to wheat ingestion or even wheat inhalation (respiratory allergy) causing baker's asthma or rhinitis (hay fever). [*12]

Non-Celiac Gluten Sensitivity (NCGS) is when an individual has a hard time digesting gluten. The immune system does not produce antibodies against the wheat gluten. This means it is not an autoimmune disease. However, the individual affected by NCGS will suffer from a wide range of intestinal symptoms like **bloating, gas, diarrhea, and stomach pain** immediately after eating gluten. [*3,53] They may also suffer **fatigue, headache, bone or joint pain, mood disorders, and skin manifestations** such as **eczema, itches, or rashes**. Even more interesting is that the presence of antigliadin IgG has been reported in up to 50% of the NCGS individuals, while antigliadin IgA antibodies rarely occur (7%). [*17,18,57]

You just want to know better so you could make better choices while maintaining your health. I would like to add a few more points:

a. Gluten is the protein part in the wheat grains family. However, we know of individuals who will react to the **oligosaccharides particles** in wheat and other grains even on rice and quinoa. The osmotic effect in the intestinal lumen will increase **gas production** from bacterial fermentation which will affect your gut flora.

[*9,37,40,63] This means that you can be negative on a food allergy test on gluten, but you feel much better when you avoid eating gluten. In such cases, a low FODMAP diet (fermentable, oligo-, di-, monosaccharides, and polyols) will be more helpful while supporting your gut flora.

b. As was discussed before, we have four different types of gliadin peptides epitopes: alpha, beta, gamma, and omega. Most labs will measure only the **Alpha-Gliadin** antibodies, but not the **Beta, Gamma, and Omega-Gliadin**. More so, most labs will not test for the **Glutenin** component, which will trigger the immune system and unfortunately, not all people will respond to the alpha-gliadin. In fact, studies show that only 50% will respond to the alpha-gliadin but not to the other gliadins and glutenin epitopes. [*6,15,24,31,45,70]

c. Gluten – **may NOT be the only food that you can be sensitive or allergic to.** Something else could be leading to unexplained weight gain.

d. Gluten can create a structural destruction mainly on the intestinal villi that can lead to infection and inflammation, and still not be celiac.

You can guess, though, it is better to TEST which foods you are sensitive or allergic to.

As you already understand, clinical symptoms vary and can be presented differently among different individuals. Some will experience extreme weight loss and some will experience weight gain. Some will have diarrhea and others constipation. Some will have stomach pain and others joint pain or both. Some will be bloated and vomit and some will not. Removing gluten from your diet will be the first step towards healing, but not the only step. As you can already see, gluten can create far more damage that will be needed to address later on in life.

If you find yourself challenged with weight gain or difficulties in losing weight, I would suggest you start with a food allergy test before adopting any nutritional programs. Diets that aren't right for you may make you frustrated, restricted, and unhealthy.

ANTIBODIES - THE IMMUNE SYSTEM RESPONSE TO YOUR FOOD ALLERGIES AND SENSITIVES

Kelly, a busy mother of three, is a 34-year-old female who joined my "Gain Health Lose Weight" program four years ago. She is 5 feet, 4 inches and at that time weighed 136 pounds. She did not work and she exercised by going to a spinning class three times a week. Her goal was to lose 4-8 pounds in less than two months. I suspected food allergies, gut challenges, and hormonal imbalances after going through an initial analysis with her. At that time, she couldn't afford food allergy testing, so we began with an elimination diet. Kelly followed it to some extent and lost some weight, but the minute she went back to her normal eating habits, she regained all her weight back and even gained four extra pounds. She was frustrated and I was too. I did not hear from her for three years and I wondered what happened to her.

Three years later, she came back. This time her weight was up to 148 pounds. She was exhausted, low in energy, had sleep apnea, and suffered rashes and itching all over her body. She was also moody and ready to start antidepressant medications. This time she agreed to do the food allergy tests. Results came back positive. She was sensitive to wheat, gluten, some beans, eggs, and dairy. Kelly's reaction to the results was, "But I eat 2 or 3 yogurts every day! I thought the Probiotic in it was good for me." **Ironically, the food you like the most is often the food you are sensitive to.** Kelly changed her diet, nourished her body with key nutrients and food supplements, and supported her damaged intestine tissues so food could be digested better. In response to those changes, inflammation markers went down, sleep and energy levels improved, her mood and hormones stabilized, and she lost 15 pounds. She is keeping her new weight scale following the Balance Diet.

The challenge for Kelly was not ONLY gluten. Gluten was positive, though taking gluten out of her diet could not fully support her for better and balanced health. For her, it was also dairy and egg yolk that stimulated her immune system and damaged her small intestine's villi, which lead to a leaky gut condition, nutrient deficiencies, hormonal imbalances, moodiness, sleep apnea and unwanted weight gain. Her weight was the only symptom she noticed and could associate with her body challenges. The root cause for her unexplained weight gain was **delayed food reaction** and the negative vicious cycle that comes with it.

What Is the Difference in the Immunologic Reactions?

There are two known major paths that your immune system can take when it recognizes a certain food as an invader: the **acute or immediate reaction** and the **delayed hypersensitivity reaction.** These responses are further classified into four types. Types I, (immediate) type II, III and IV (delayed). On an **acute reaction (type I),** the immune system will produce the antibody IgE within 30 minutes to 3 hours from ingesting the "agent" that was introduced into the body.

Most immediate reactions are so fast that individuals can easily identify the cause of their reactions and eliminate it in the future to protect themselves. The agent could be gluten or any other food. Surprisingly, even romaine lettuce could be recognized as a pathogen by your immune system, which will activate the production of the antibody IgE. In such cases, it could impact your weight. Antigens will bind to IgE antibodies, which attach to the surface of the mast cell or the basophil and cause the release of chemical mediators such as histamine and eosinophilic chemotactic factor. Thus, the individual will experience a variety of allergy symptoms depending on the location of the mast cell, and inflammation that will cause tissue damage over time. The symptoms of acute reactions are varied and could be: **eczema, redness and small blistering, bronchitis, asthma, coughing, sneezing, diarrhea, intestinal mucosa, intestinal spasm, nutrients malabsorption, inflammation, colic, vomiting, spitting, joint pain, hives, itching, or burning and swelling of the skin. Headaches, loss of memory, and difficulty concentrating** may also be symptoms of a food allergy. In extreme cases, some people may experience **anaphylactic shock.**

On a **delayed hypersensitivity** reaction (type II), different immunoglobulin class antibodies will be produced. With such conditions, the **IgG and IgM antibody**-mediated with symptoms two hours to up to 72 hours after the offending food has been ingested. The degree and severity of symptoms vary based on the genetic makeup of the individual. Delayed food sensitivity is associated with a multitude of disorders, such as **multiple sclerosis, autism, rheumatoid arthritis, migraines, mood swings, fatigue, intestinal upset, joint pain, high blood pressure and attention disorders,** which affect an estimated 40% of the population. [33,44,50,51] This is BIG!

To make it more challenging, the **IgG and IgM antibodies** will activate **the complement system** (type III and IV). The antibodies bind directly with the particular food (not the mast cells) which enter the bloodstream. This process enhances the ability of the immune system antibodies to clear, attack, and kill the pathogen's plasma membrane – the "invader agent," releasing protease, mast cells, and vasoactive amines that promote inflammation. That leads to tissue damage which will eventually affect your weight. In type IV, there is the presence of granulomatous tissue rejection due to macrophage stimulation. This increases the production of chemical agents, such as histamines, cytokines, lymphokines, and interferons as well. This process can last between 60 to 90 days and up to 15 weeks, after the allergen agent was introduced. **The symptoms for delayed reaction** could be **gastrointestinal complaints** such as **nausea, vomiting, diarrhea** and/or constipation, stomachache, irritable bowel, Crohn's disease, ulcerative colitis; skin complaints: itching, eczema, hives, acne (in adults), and even psoriasis; joint and muscle complaints ranging from atypical pains to rheumatoid arthritis, swelling, fibromyalgia, headache, migraine, chronic fatigue, asthma, chronic rhinitis or sinusitis, pre-menstrual syndrome, hypoglycemia, depression, anxiety, sleeping disorders, blurring of vision due to retinitis, ringing in the ears, cold and flu symptoms, heart palpitations, arrhythmia, increased heart rate, and unexplained salt/water retention due to the immune system complex activity.

Food allergens must be present in the body to start these immune system reactions. These bio-chemical reactions could affect any of your body systems from skin through: **GI mucosal, cardiovascular system, respiratory tract, hormones, and brain dysfunctions.** If you suspect gluten sensitivity, celiac, or food allergy, I highly recommend you get tested and heal the tissues that have been damaged.

Suggested Tests:

a. Gluten allergy or Celiac: You may want to consider taking the genetic gene blood test called **the human leukocyte antigen (HLA) class II alleles**: HLA-DQ 2 and HLA-8. HLA is a type of molecule that presented against gluten antigens to T-cells which reduce the tissue damage. Studies show that 95% of individuals with celiac disease will have HLA-DQ2 and 5% of HLA-DQ8. [51,60] More interesting is the fact that 73% of patients with insulin-dependent diabetes mellitus were found to carry either one of the two HLA-DQ [22,50] This also occurs in individuals with auto-immune thyroiditis (Hashimoto's disease) [44,52] and unexplained iron deficiency anemia. [33]

b. **IgE and IgG Antibodies blood test.** These tests measure your sensitivity to certain foods from an antibody-mediated immune response. Some labs will test a group of 96, 144, or 250 foods either by "finger stick," blood spots that need to be collected and shipped directly to the laboratory in a pre-paid envelope, or by a professional lab drawing the blood from a vein.

c. **Skin tests** - Scratch test and intradermal test.

If you are not tested and the "harmful" food is not eliminated, there is no way your body will be able to maintain a healthy and balanced weight.

GRAINS ARE NO LONGER HEALTHY - THE GLYPHOSATE CONNECTION

The seeds of grains are sprayed with herbicides, fungicides, and insecticides containing the toxic active ingredient glyphosate found in the herbicide Roundup- (a common product that is used to kill weeds). The chemical glyphosate is spread 7 to 10 days before harvest to dry the plant and to ease the harvest process. According to the US Department of Agriculture, as of 2012, 99% of durum wheat, 97% of spring wheat, and 61% of winter wheat has been treated with herbicides. This is an increase from 88% of durum wheat, 91% of spring wheat and 47% of winter wheat in 1998.

These chemicals are continuing to act in our body. It disrupts the seven steps of a metabolic route called **shikimate pathway,** found and used in the beneficial gut microbes (also like probiotic) which is responsible for synthesis of amino acids. Glyphosate also inhibits the **cytochrome P450** (CYP) enzymes produced by the gut microbiome. CYP enzymes are critical to human biology because they detoxify the multitude of foreign chemical compounds, xenobiotics, that we are exposed to in our modern environment. [60]

The study also reflects on how the usage of glyphosate on wheat in the U.S. has risen sharply in the last decade, in step with the sharp rise in the incidence of Celiac disease, intestinal infections and Thyroid cancer. [*75]

Unfortunately, most grains carry the chemical glyphosate which may affect our hormonal balances, damage our intestines, and create systemic inflammation. These effects increase risk of experiencing a gene expression in a form of "labeled" disease based on the gene blueprints we born with as well as nutrient deficiencies and weight gain.

Don't save, spend the extra money, test yourself for a delayed food sensitivity. Balance your body with proper nutrients that fits your needs.

If you are NOT found to have any food sensitivity, my best recommendations are:

a. Consume organic and non-GMO grains if possible.

b. Consume low glycemic gluten or gluten free grains

c. Make sure you consume grains in moderation

NUTRIENT IMBALANCES

As strange as it sounds, many studies will point out that overweight and obese individuals are nutritionally depleted. [1,28,57] They are shown to have lower levels of B vitamins, A, C, D, folate, calcium, magnesium, selenium, zinc, and chromium, as well as lower levels of anti-oxidants and certain fat-soluble vitamins. These are all negative contributors to nutrient deficiencies which leads to weight gain. [15,56] In many cases, the cause for weight gain is the inadequate consumption of fruits and vegetables on daily basis. Moreover, over consumption of low quality of nutrients, lack of dense foods, high intake of "empty" calories from fats, sugar, sweetened beverages, and processed foods can add up as the reason of weight gain. These factors are associated with nutritional depletion and, in extreme cases, undernourishment. As a result, production of higher bio-waste toxins keeps this vicious cycle going and leads to further weight gain and development of metabolic diseases like high blood pressure, high cholesterol, and high blood sugar levels, and inflammation. [10,24,47] Nutrient depletion can lead to more stress on your body's systems which will slow down any healing process and will prevent your desire lose weight. **Micronutrients are**

essential for our day-to-day, mind-body-spirt performance and healthy body weight.

Gluten-free grains will NOT stop nutritional deficiencies. If you are found to have gluten sensitivity. In fact, it will lead to further depletion of vitamins, minerals, and fibers. In most cases, it will keep your weight the same or you will gain more.

At this point, you may want to rethink your gluten-free diet options. The correct question is: **Do you need to be on a gluten-free diet for medical reasons or not?** If yes, then learn how to eat properly. Support your body with appropriate food and food supplements so you do NOT deplete yourself. If you do not have a medical reason, then you want to continue eating grains in moderation as part of a healthy diet.

WHAT CHALLENGES DOES THE GLUTEN-FREE DIET BRING?

The actual challenge of being on a gluten-free diet if you wish to lose weight (unless you are found to be gluten sensitive or allergic), is the quantities and the quality of the food you should eat. Most individuals on the Balance Diet (which I'll go over it in details later in this book), admit that the true challenge is eating higher quantities than they used to eat, as well as the effort it takes to prepare and eat high quality and quantities of foods. We must listen to our gut's ability to digest grains and lower the risk for chronic inflammation of the intestinal mucosa. We must balance our nutrient deficiencies.

Jack, one of my clients, is a good example of a health-conscious person who gained almost 17 pounds in less than 12 months. He just couldn't understand what went wrong. Jack came to my clinic to lose weight three years ago. At the time, he was 45 year-old man with four children. He worked in the finance industry in the Bay area. Jack is 6 feet tall, 232 pounds, rides his bicycle 30 miles twice a week, is a vegetarian and ate a healthy diet on a daily basis. On the initial evaluation, it was clear he is not digesting his food properly. Since he became a vegetarian, he noticed that he had even worse smelling gas, bloating, diarrhea, constipation, and sometimes nausea and fatigue. On his vegetarian diet, he consumed 1-2 cups of beans daily (different types) and at least 1 cup of grains, including quinoa and millet (both considered gluten-free grains). To improve digestion, Jack learned how to soak and sprout his grains and beans. This method, helps to reduce plant based toxins and ease digestion. We also, modified food quantities, and food quality which gradually closed the nutrients gap, energy levels increased, and therefore, he could experience weight loss. The fact that he couldn't digest plant fibers lead him to a nutrient depletion and weight gain. Supporting the root cause made a shift in his life.

THE EFFECT ON YOUR B VITAMINS

Carbohydrates are our primary energy source. Cutting back on gluten and whole grains may reduce your vitamin B intake which will increase your risk of chronic disease. Vitamin B's are a group of water soluble-vitamins that are crucial for cell metabolism. There are eight known Vitamin B's: B1 (thiamine), Vitamin B2 (riboflavin), Vitamin B3 (niacin), Vitamin B5 (pantothenic acid), Vitamin B6 (pyridoxine, or pyridoxamine), Vitamin B7 Vitamin B9 (folate) and Vitamin B12. This group of eight vitamins plays a vital role in our oxidation of fatty acids and carbohydrates pathways. Some are involved in our amino acids, lipids, and cholesterol metabolism. Some synthesize our neurotransmitters and hemoglobin production and some are critical co-factors to vitamins A, C, D, E, and K.

VITAMIN B DEFICIENCIES

When you are on a gluten-free diet, you give up a great source of vitamin B - the grains. Those who are diagnosed with Celiac disease or have high sensitivities to gluten are at an increased risk of developing nutritional deficiencies of B vitamins, calcium, vitamin D, iron, zinc, magnesium, or fibers. [14,22,31,54] A 10 year study published in 2002 concluded that celiac patients living on a gluten-free diet for several years had higher total plasma of homocysteine levels than the general population. This is an indicator of poor vitamin status. In accordance, the plasma levels of folate and pyridoxal 5-phosphate (the active form of vitamin B-6) were low in 37% and 20%, respectively, and accounted for 33% of the variation of the total plasma homocysteine level (P < 0.008). The mean daily intakes of folate and vitamin B-12, but not of vitamin B-6, were significantly lower in celiac patients than in the control group, apart from the intake of vitamin B-6. The study concluded that half of the adult celiac patients who were carefully treated with a gluten-free diet for several years showed signs of a poor vitamin status. [* 14,22,23,31,53]

In fact, research suggested that **low B12 or high homocysteine markers are the first sign of malabsorption**. Other studies demonstrate that 20-38% of celiac patients have nutritional deficiencies and lack of dietary fiber as well as low mineral and vitamin levels. [*9,26,27,30] Individuals experiencing low levels of the nutrients mentioned above are prone to intestinal malabsorption. They are also predisposed to a mucosal state of the upper intestinal tract that may lead to intestinal dysbiosis, leaky gut, and/or gut inflammation, atrophic gastritis, or hypochlorhydria (which is low stomach acid), pernicious anemia, and autoimmune conditions. Taking medications, drinking alcohol, and exposure to nitrous oxide will affect the nutritional deficiencies process as well, whether or not you are on gluten-free diet.

If you are choosing a gluten-free diet as non-celiac person, you are increasing your chance to develop vitamin B deficiencies. You want to make sure you are using products that are enriched or fortified with B vitamins and iron like most gluten and wheat flour. Gluten-free flour is NOT (yet), enriched or fortified. You may think that you get the nutrients based on your experience with gluten flour, but it's not the case with all gluten-free products.

Make sure you consume or supplement these key nutrients on a daily basis. Remember, **amaranth, spelt, rice flour, or any gluten-free starches like tapioca or potato simply don't have the fiber and nutrients of whole grains.**

Taking a B vitamin supplement can help close the nutrient gap. The recommended dose depends on your blood tests results; however, the suggested dose is 1-2mg per day. When you supplement with these nutrients, you want to take some extra caution. **Toxicity can develop if you overdose.** Taking more vitamin B6 than needed, for example, could affect your nerves and even damage nerve signals. Excess of pyridoxine B6 can be presented with a painful numbness and tingling in the hands and feet. Ataxia (loss of coordination in body movement), painful skin lesions, nausea, heartburn, and photosensitivity can be present too. If this is the case, you want to stop all sources of pyridoxine.

Consult a doctor or a professional nutritionist. Do not skimp on additional blood tests to measure your nutrient levels. When you reach the normal range, stop taking the supplement or reduce the dosage.

POTENTIAL IRON ANEMIA

A high rate of Anemia is presented among individuals with Celiac disease who are on a gluten-free diet. Iron plays a crucial role in the heme group of hemoglobin to transport oxygen. Anemia is a condition that results from a deficiency in the size or number of red blood cells or the amount of hemoglobin in these cells. There are many reasons why people are low in iron and ferritin levels. However, the most common reason is due to iron, folate, and/or vitamin B12 deficiency. In people with Celiac disease (most likely among people with gluten sensitivity as well) the damage on the intestinal villi is one of many reasons for developing anemia. Iron from food is absorbed mainly in the upper intestines, the same part of the intestines damaged by gluten. Low stomach acid can constitute to low iron levels as well, even if the intestinal villi are not yet damaged. [*11,18,37]

If you are taking acid blocking agents like Omerprazole, Protonicx, Prilosec, or Zantec for the treatment of reflux or ulcers you, most likely will face low stomach acid levels which will affect your iron levels. [*2,40,55,58]

Another aspect of iron deficiencies is related to a low level of lactoferrin, a protein and antioxidant used by the immune system to protect us from intestinal bacterial, fungal, parasite, and viral infections. These include: Listeria, Staphylococcus, Salmonella, Clostridium, and Escherichia coli. Lactoferrin helps regulate the absorption of iron in the intestine and the delivery of iron to the cells. Individuals with GI challenges, regardless of a gluten-free diet, will face low Lactoferrin and low Iron levels. [*4,1238,39]

Studies also indicate that low levels of Lactoferrin will affect your body's ability to reduce fat at the cellular level. Lactoferrin works by inhibiting fat synthesis and stimulating liberation of stored body fat (a process called lipolysis). [*8,35,45] More than that, high levels of Lactoferrin are associated with lower Body Mass Index (BMI), lower fasting triglyceride (blood fat), and glucose concentrations. [*7,41,42]

Anemia leads to oxygen deficiency, which in turn can reduce the body's ability to generate energy, cell growth, reproduction, and support for the immune system, which in turn can cause a cyclic state of healing inhibition.

Aside from gluten induced damage, iron deficiency can occur in menstruating women with mild to heavy periods. Iron deficiency can also happen when there is slow but steady blood loss. This can occur in a hidden manner (occult blood loss), or it can be more obvious as in the case of hemorrhoids. So, if you are a menstruating woman, on a gluten-free diet, restricting your caloric intake, or going to the gym at least 3 times a week to lose weight, you face an increased risk for developing anemia.

When you are on a gluten-free diet, most likely your iron levels will decline. Simple blood test results will give you the needed information to address any deficiencies either by adding foods, food supplements, or a combination of both, so you can prevent any further stress on your body.

Gluten-free Sources for Iron

- Red meat, pork, lamb, liver, other organ meats
- Fish, clams, mussels, oysters, sardines, anchovies
- Poultry, chicken, duck, turkey, liver (especially dark meat)
- Flour made from soybeans, chickpeas (garbanzo beans), buckwheat, quinoa, amaranth, or teff
- Legumes - lentils, chickpeas, green peas, kidney beans, lima beans, pinto beans, black-eyed peas
- Pumpkin seeds, sesame seeds, cashews, almonds
- Dark leafy greens (spinach, Swiss chard, Boc Choy, turnip, kale, collard, Brussels Sprouts, broccoli)
- Apricots, prunes, raisins
- Gluten-free pasta, cereal, or bread fortified with iron

Gluten-free Grain Sources of Iron (1 cup of raw grain 13)

- Amaranth 15 mg
- Teff 14.7 mg
- Sorghum 8.4 mg
- Quinoa 7.7 mg
- GF Oats 7.4 mg
- Millet 6 mg
- Buckwheat 3.7 mg
- Brown Rice 2.7
- White Rice 1.5 mg

POTENTIAL FOLATE FOR VITAMIN B12 ANEMIA

As mentioned, Anemia is the name for the iron-deficiency that affects our red blood cell sizes or the amount of hemoglobin they contain. However, anemia can be developed by a deficiency of folate and or vitamin B12 too. [*5,38]

If you have <u>Iron-deficiency anemia</u> you will face extreme **fatigue, weakness, brittle nails,** and **decreased appetite**. If you deal with <u>Folate-deficiency Anemia</u> on top of the iron-deficiency symptoms, you may have **ringing in the ears, cracked lips, sore tongue, irregular heartbeat and chest pains.** If you have Vitamin B12-deficiency Anemia you may also experience **depression, numbness or tingling** in the hands and feet, **muscle weakness, lack of coordination, and balance problems** on top of the folate deficiency symptoms. Folate is crucial for normal red blood cell formation, for the creation of nucleic acids including the DNA and for the amino acids synthesis. [*19,20,33]

B12 anemia can indicate challenges to your digestive tract in absorbing B12. We need B12 for the self-production of red blood cells as well as for supporting our nervous system.

In cases where the stomach lining is slow or cannot produce intrinsic factor (a chemical produced by the stomach lining binding with B12 in the small intestine) the challenges are greater to maintain B12 levels. Individuals with Chron's disease, which is a chronic inflammatory disease, will face low B12 levels as well. [*3,51]

If you are facing any type of anemia, it will not help your goal to lose weight. Only after balancing and addressing anemia, will you begin seeing changes to your weight.

Most gluten-free flours, breads, pastas, and cold cereal products are not enriched with folate or iron. As with whole grains, the natural folate is not found. Based on the 2010 Dietary Guidelines adults need 400 mcg of folate, which is equal to nearly 7 cups of raw spinach or 4 cups of fortified breakfast cereal. Women that are planning to become pregnant will need about 200 mcg more, which takes you up to 600 mcg per day. **When was the last time you had 7 cups of spinach in one single day?**

If you are on a gluten-free diet, you want to choose foods that will provide sufficient iron, folate, and vitamin B12 to prevent any deficiencies in the future. Choose gluten-free whole grains that can provide you with this valued nutrient - folate. Quinoa, asparagus, beans, and vegetables are some of the food choices you can add to your daily food intake to meet the needed requirements (as long you are not sensitive to any of those foods).

Gluten-free Source of Folate

- Animal protein including poultry, pork, liver, and shellfish
- Garbanzo beans (chickpea)/Hummus or non-GMO corn flour
- Pinto beans, lentils, great northern beans, and kidney beans
- Soy beans (edamame)
- Asparagus, beets, broccoli, Brussels sprouts, avocado, collard greens, corn, green peas, romaine lettuce, and bok-choy
- Bananas, oranges, pineapple, strawberries, melons, and tomatoes

Gluten-free Grain Source of Folate

- Enriched gluten-free breads, cereals and pasta
- Amaranth grains or flour
- Bean flours
- Garbanzo beans or flour
- Soy beans or flour
- Corn meal

- Ground flax
- Millet grains or flour
- Quinoa grains or flour
- Rice grains or flour
- Teff grains or flour
- Wild rice

Gluten-free Source of Vitamin B12

- Red meat, liver (beef), lamb, and turkey
- Chicken
- Fish, shellfish (scallops, shrimps), mackerel, crustaceans (crab), salmon, sardines, tuna and cod
- Diary: milk, yogurt, cheese
- Eggs
- Organic, non-GMO, Fortified Soy Products
- Mushrooms

Plant based foods that have been fortified with B12 like rice, soy beverages, plant derived meat, ready to eat breakfast gluten-free cereal, and nutritional yeast can be additional sources of vitamin B12. You need to review the quality of your food sources and the quality of the added vitamin B12 sources, sugars, and fats.

If you choose animal based protein as your healthy source of B12, choose: **organic, grass fed, hormone-free and antibiotic-free sources** (beef, chicken, or turkey). As for fish, you probably want to choose **wild-caught fish** over farm raised fish.

Unbalanced nutrients such as deficiencies or elevation of any of these nutrients will affect your overall health. It doesn't matter if you are on a gluten-free diet or not.

If your goal is to lose weight, you want to balance your body with enough nutrients to support all bio-mechanism for optimal health. Remember, once you are nutrient depleted your chances to lose weight are slim. Therefore, you want to include high quality of grains (gluten-free or not), protein, fats, fruits, and vegetables that will provide you with all eight B vitamins, and many more nutrient requirements to balance your metabolism so you can lose weight easily.

THE EFFECT ON YOUR VITAMIN D – CALCIUM LEVELS

Vitamin D is crucial for our optimum function. Vitamin D is involved in our calcium absorption and our bone health because it promotes the minerals and growth factors to our bones. Vitamin D is involved in our brain function, cardiovascular health, and the immune system. It activates killer T-cells to protect our cells from infections, bacterial activity, modulation, and expression of genes, which regulate cell proliferation for apoptosis and WBC differentiations. Vitamin D receptors are crucial in maintaining the integrity of the intestinal mucosal barrier and the pancreatic enzymes. [*34,36,43,44,46] Healthy levels of vitamin D are critical to our health and to stabilize our weight, in particular if you are on a gluten-free diet. Some studies even suggest that low levels of vitamin D are associated with weight gain and at the same time may predispose you to fat accumulation. [*6,17,32,52]

The most important action of vitamin D is to increase the active absorption of calcium. Seventy percent (70%) of Celiac sensitive individuals are suffering from a reduced bone mineral density. Low levels of vitamin D consequently affects your levels of calcium. Severe cases of vitamin D deficiency may lead to poorly mineralized bones, osteomalacia (soft bones) or rickets due to low levels of calcium absorption. Even if you supplement yourself with calcium only 10-15% of dietary calcium is absorbed (compared to 30-40% in healthy individuals) when vitamin D is low. The assumption is that people on a gluten-free diet will deplete levels of vitamin D and calcium levels which will affect their bone mineral density over time. Studies show that even if you are on a strict gluten-free diet, supplementing your body with vitamin D and calcium over a one -year period, bone mineral density will still become low compared to those who are not on a gluten diet.[13,21]

In addition, poor calcium absorption will lead to increased levels of the parathyroid hormone, which helps to metabolize and regulate calcium in the body. With low vitamin D, bone metabolism will be affected and thus reduce the active calcium absorption. The parathyroid hormone (PTH), which functions as a calcium sensor, will increase the secretion of calcitriol which stimulates the calcium absorption from the gut, bone, and kidneys. This will activate bone resorption. When calcium levels rise, the feedback mechanism will sense the PTH to turn and drop off the secretion of calcitriol. If that does not happen, then the thyroid gland will secrete calcitonin, which can block bone calcium resorption, helping to keep serum calcium levels in the normal range. [59,60] Most individuals on a gluten-free diet were found to be low in vitamin D, parathyroid hormone level was significantly higher, and bone mineral density (BMD) was significantly lower.[50]

We can absorb only about 30% of calcium coming from food. This depends on the type of food we eat as well as the amount we consume. In fact, 72% of our calcium will come from milk and milk products. The remaining calcium sources come from vegetables (7%), grains (5%), legumes (4%), fruits (3%), meat, poultry, fish (3%), eggs (2%), and other foods (3%).[16] The absorption of calcium percentages is much higher if you eat green vegetables like arugula, bok choy, broccoli, chard, and kale. If you eat more food that carries high levels of the binding calcium compounds like oxalic acid and phytic acid, your calcium levels are unlikely to rise as much as you expected. Foods like spinach, collard greens, sweet potatoes, rhubarb, beans, seeds, nuts, whole-grain products, wheat bran, and soy isolates which carry high levels of oxalic acid and phytic acid.

High levels of protein, sodium, potassium, and caffeine (from coffee and tea) intake will increase calcium excretion and reduce the absorption. [*29,59,60]

The Institute of Medicine recommends a daily calcium intake of 1,000 mg (milligrams) for men and women up to age 50. Women over age 50 and men over age 70 should increase their intake to 1,200-1,500 mg daily. As for vitamin D, the recommended intake is 600 to 800 IU (International Units) each day.

On a gluten-free diet, most individuals will not eat enough vegetables, legumes, and fruits. Their gluten-free grains are not diverse and nourishing. In most cases, gluten will not be the only food they eliminate from their diet. Some will also eliminate dairy and/or eggs, which again, reduces their vitamin D and calcium levels. Supplements are essential, but not the only option. We need to eat enough to provide our body with a full spectrum of nutrients for a Balanced life. We just can't ignore it. Vitamin D and calcium are vital nutrients for our health and our weight.

Gluten-free Source of Calcium

- <u>Dairy products:</u> milk, yogurt, cheeses, and buttermilk
- <u>Vegetables:</u> Dark green, leafy vegetables as broccoli, collards, kale, mustard greens, turnip greens, bok choy, spinach, arugula, cilantro, dill, parsley, turnip greens, rhubarb, collard greens, okra, peas, brussels sprouts, and chinese cabbage
- <u>Fish:</u> Bony salmon, sardines, and shellfish will increase your weekly calcium intake. Aim to have two portions of bony fish per week (1 portion = 100 gram or 3 oz). The bones contain the most calcium levels.
- <u>Nuts and seeds</u> like almonds, Brazil nuts, chia, and sesame seeds. Sprinkle your seeds over your salads, protein, and fats to enrich your calcium levels.
- <u>Beans</u> and legumes

Calcium supplements are a must in some cases, though you want to monitor your calcium levels. Increased intake of calcium can lead to confusion, constipation, and fatigue. It can also lead to low levels of magnesium and iron, irritability, and kidney damage. If this happens to you, stop your calcium intake immediately. If you are supplementing with calcium, you want to make sure you are including magnesium and vitamin D.

Gluten-free Sources of Vitamin D

- Cod liver oil
- Fatty fish (mackerel, salmon, tuna, sardines, herring, shrimp)
- Milk or soy milk
- Egg yolk

The sun obviously is a great source of getting natural vitamin D and, therefore, you need to expose yourself to sunlight. Being active will support your goal to lose weight as well. However, don't let yourself fall on the extremes of either doing too much or too little. Make it fun. Walk, do gardening, do yoga, go outdoors in your backyard. . . Expose your hands and feet for about fifteen minutes a day. Eliminate the use of sunscreen or at least look for a better product that will support your body (especially with kids). Limit time spent outside. Wearing light cotton shirts instead can be helpful.

The point is clear – if you are **on a gluten-free diet, over time you will develop nutrient deficiencies.** My clinical experience is that most people are not consuming enough vegetables, fruits, nut, seeds, protein, and healthy fats to meet the daily needs of their body. **A big, nice fresh salad once or twice a day could help you close the nutrient gap.**

CELLULAR RESPIRATION AND WEIGHT GAIN CONNECTION

Maintaining a healthy body weight depends largely on how efficient your mitochondria energy production is. Mitochondria are the driving force within each cell in the body. It is a vital force for your health as well as maintaining a healthy weight. Mitochondria energy production is dependent upon nutrient levels, thyroid function, level of toxin exposure, food allergies or sensitivities, level of oxidative stress, physical activity, and genes. It could be one or a combination of these several factors which affect the body's energy production. As a result, this affects your weight regardless of whether you choose to eat gluten free grains or not.

The body's "gasoline" fuel molecule is called ATP (Adenosine Triphosphate). ATP is produced by a combination of oxygen with macro nutrient foods. It's a very complex system which involves many electrochemical stages such as the citric acid cycle, the Krebs cycle, the electron transport chain pathway, fatty acid oxidation, gluconeogenesis, and oxidative phosphorylation. These are all involved with this fascinating process to produce 1 unit of ATP molecule.

With optimum balanced mitochondria, your body will have sufficient oxygen as well as nutrients consisting of mainly proteins, fats, and carbohydrates. At this balanced level, the mitochondria will produce ATP energy. As a result, the metabolism will become more efficient while energy levels, hormones, brain and heart health will improve while a healthy weight is maintained. This energy production process is not only dependent on proteins, fats, and carbohydrates, but also upon vitamins, minerals, and amino acids such as calcium ion, glutathione, CoQ10, and more. Significant changes (excessiveness or depletion) to oxygen levels or nutrient deficiencies will create oxidative stress which slows down the body's energy production. Therefore, low energy, fatigue, memory loss, pain, and weight gain will occur. When mitochondria are working effectively, it's a clean-burning, oxygen-utilizing, metabolic engine. Otherwise, infection, dehydration, accumulation of toxins, oxidative stress, and oxidative damage will slow down energy production, which in turn affects your weight.[*4,9] Mitochondria occasionally fuse, divide and regenerate in a process called biogenesis. Biogenesis is a quality control process in case there are mitochondrial damages to create healthy mitochondria cells. This process, of course, also depends on nutrients.[*3]

Oxidation is a process where higher free radicals presented in the body compare to antioxidants. It is a chemical reaction where unstable and unpaired electrons are "homeless," looking for partner while stealing or damaging other molecules and therefore affecting normal cell functionality.[*8,12] The challenges the body faces under this oxidation process and low ATP energy production are that a greater percentage of oxidative energy will be stored as fat rather than used as energy.[*3] In many cases, it can be considered the first sign of potential long-term damage due to oxidative stress associated with: chronic degenerative diseases. Gut pathogens such as yeast overgrowth, bacteria, parasites, toxic exposure, or even over-exercising may lead to nutrient depletion and weight gain. The balance between oxidation and oxygen levels is very delicate and crucial for cellular biochemistry. This balance is dependent on nutrient intake, which is why it's so vital to eat real food every single day!

Age decreases mitochondria efficiency by 8% every 10 years and approximately by 40% in the elderly years (61-84 years of age). This happens due to mitochondrial oxidative and phosphorylation activity. These bodily reactions will affect lipid content and insulin sensitivity as well as insulin resistance. That means less energy production, more fatigue, and a slower metabolism as we age, regardless of whether or not we eat gluten or gluten-free grains. In a depleted nutrient state, the ability to lose weight also decreases. [10,11]

First, another factor to consider when discussing bodily energy production is a healthy thyroid. In a balanced environment, the thyroid gland produces the hormone T4 (thyroxine). T4 will then be converted into the active form T3 (triiodothtyonline). Then T3 turns on the ATP inside of each cell, supporting your cellular mitochondria energy production. The thyroid glands are challenged because of one of the following reasons: the thyroid can't produce enough or is producing too much T4. Second, the lack of vitamins or minerals to support the enzymes and co-factors needed to activate the ATP molecule in each cell, auto-immune disease and lastly, the accumulation of too many toxins or there is too much oxidative stress. When one or a combination of these factors exist inside your body, energy production becomes compromised. You feel fatigued, your memory declines, and body temperature fluctuates. This triggers most people to eat more carbs and sweets which results in weight gain. [2,5,6]

When a person begins a calorie restricted diet, even if it's a gluten-free diet, his or her metabolic rate will decline. This means the expected weight loss is almost always less than the effort needed to keep up the body's energy needs. The quality and the quantity of the food choices made will support a healthy and balanced energy production as well as a balanced weight. The most critical factors to maintaining a healthy weight are nutrition and energy homeostasis. If your body can't convert foods into energy, there will be mitochondrial dysfunction. In extreme cases, this leads to anorexia, starvation, and cachexia (extreme condition of weight loss which involves muscle atrophy, fatigue, loss of appetite, and weakness). The bottom line is, in most cases, you will begin gaining weight due to a slower metabolic rate when going on a calorie restricted diet. [7,12]

Comprehensive evaluation and testing of your nutritional needs by a professional nutritionist will lead to designing a specific diet and curing potential nutrient deficiencies. This is made possible by using real foods, food supplements, increasing quality of foods (organic, non-GMO, fresh, local), and increasing meal frequency altogether. Over time, this will support your mitochondria energy production, leading to a much healthier weight! [8]

THE GUT-WEIGHT GAIN CONNECTION

Whether you are on a gluten or gluten-free diet, vegan, Paleo, or Mediterranean diet, if your gut is not properly digesting, absorbing, assimilating, and eliminating the foods you are eating, chances are you will gain weight. It's a long process that involves mechanical steps and chemical reactions which release nutrients from the food you eat into your body. The quality, the quantities, and the diversity of your gut bacteria will affect your weight. This is the reason why we want to have healthy gut, but first we need to understand why the gut micro-biome is maybe the most significant factor towards achieving optimum health and weight. [*26]

In our gut, we have about 10 trillion micro-organisms consisting of viruses, bacteria, fungi, and parasites. There are ten times more gut bacteria than all of the human cells combined entirely. In fact, there are over 400 known gut bacterial species. [*28] The health of your gut reflects your overall health and equals a healthy and balanced weight.

Each person has his or her own composition of gut microbes as part of the core set of micro-organisms common to us all. [*18,27] The human microbiota is established early in life, starting in the womb and through the birth canal (compared to those born through a Caesarean procedure). Your gut microbe can be affected by food, exposure to environmental toxins, bio-toxins, age, geographical location, food supplemental intake, and drugs or medication. [*4]

Your gut microbiome is involved in the metabolism of complex carbohydrates. Humans simply don't have the enzymes to break down complex carbohydrates and thus are completely dependent on the gut microbe to do this "work" for them. Other gut microbes will produce vitamins and minerals such as biotin and vitamin B12, niacin, pyridoxine, and vitamin K. [*14]They will also produce short chain fatty acids (SCFAs) which regulate the immune system. [*13] These other gut microbes also protect us against invaders, inflammation, infections, allergens, and antibodies that can lead to autoimmune diseases. [*12]The gut micro-biome supports us through liver detoxification. It also supports the nervous system and brain function. There is no denying that the gut micro-biome contributes to your overall health and weight.

There are two main phyla ("groups") of gut bacteria species: The Firmicutes and the Bacteroidetes. Studies document a correlation between obesity and changes in the ratio between these two groups of gut bacteria, more specifically in favor of the Firmicutes. Since these groups of species ferment fibers more effectively, people will get more calories out of their foods due the higher quantity of this species in the gut. That fact alone could increase weight by 10 to 15 pounds over the period of 1 year, even without eating a single bite! [*20]

Additionally, studies show a direct correlation between gut flora and weight. Overweight and obese people have less healthy bacteria compared to lean people, not to mention they also have less gut bacteria diversity. [*17,25,29] Other studies found that overweight and obese people will accumulate lipid during adipogenesis due to lower levels of healthy bacteria, specifically bacteriodes. [*30]

As you already know, intestinal microbes encompass beneficial and harmful bacteria. Both will create metabolite toxins, but only an amount the liver and kidneys can handle. When the microbes are out of proportion, these toxins will build up, leading to inflammation of the gut's intestinal lining, which over time will create tissue damage. One disorder associated with these bio-toxins is a **Candida infection** that can attach to the intestinal walls, causing food allergies, nutrient deficiencies, weakened immune system, and eventual weight gain. [17] Other disorders associated with these bio-toxins are gut disybiosis, Small Intestinal Bacterial Overgrowth (SIBO), leaky gut, Irritable Bowel Syndrome (IBS), Crohn's disease, and ulcerative colitis. [10,11,24]

Some bacteria toxins such as clostridia and 3-(3-hydroxyphenyl)-3-hydroxypropionic acid (HPHPA) show an indirect relationship to weight gain due to IgA response. This type of bacteria toxicity can even inhibit neurotransmitters in the brain, including the conversion of dopamine into norepinephrine. This can lead to moodiness, depression, bipolar disorder, autism, and cravings for sweets. These can all lead to weight gain. [22]

All foods are digested and metabolized by gut flora. [21] Unfortunately, most foods are refined carbohydrates which have limited to no benefit to the gut microbe. High-fat, sugary, and processed food are absorbed in the upper part of the gut. This means fewer minerals and vitamins reach the large intestinal tract, creating a reduced biodiversity of the gut micro-biome. This creates nutrient deficiencies which leads to weight gain. [2,3,5] You need **enzymes, gastric and stomach juices, hydrochloric acids, and electrolytes** to break down food to maintain this amazing gut orchestra synchronicity!

Excessive usage of antibiotics, either directly through medications or indirectly through eating meat that is bombarded with antibiotics, is another adverse contributor to an unhealthy gut microbe and weight gain. Studies show a link between antibiotics and gut bacteria composition which affects the ability to break down nutrients properly. The result is the activation of genes which turn carbohydrates into short chain fatty acids. This activates genes related to lipid conversion in the liver. In layman's terms, these shifts in molecular pathways enable fat build-up. [1,16]

Zonulin is an inflammatory protein secreted in the intestinal mucosa. It is a healthy protected mechanism if found in small amounts. Zonulin is responsible for opening the "intestinal doors" - the tight junctions between cells - so that contaminated foods or harmful bacteria flushes out. Once the pathogen is gone, Zonulin levels will drop down, and the intestinal junctions will close.

With high levels of Zonulin the "door is left open." Gut bacteria and toxins will leak into the bloodstream. These macro-molecules will activate the immune system, damaging the natural way our bodies achieve and maintain healthy gut bacteria. High levels of Zonulin are associated with inflammatory bowel disease, Celiac disease, food allergies, irritable bowel syndrome, autoimmune diseases, obesity, and metabolic disease. Most interestingly, gliadin – the protein in wheat, oat, rye and barley – can activate the self-production of Zonulin in people that are allergic to it. When that happens, it harms the intestinal hyper-permeability, creating what's known as "leaky gut" and a vicious cycle of nutrient depletion that leads to immune response and weight gain. [9,15,19,23] The message here is clear: If you are sensitive or allergic to gliadin (the protein found in wheat), you want to AVOID it altogether while taking care of your gut. If not, studies show that different whole grains (vs. refined), in small amounts, will keep your Zonulin levels in control and protect your gut bacteria. [7,8]

I'd like you to meet Tim who is 42 years old and overweight. He suffered for the last 5 years with Rheumatoid arthritis, high CRP (4.5), digestive challenges including constipation and diarrhea in rotation, bloating gasses with excessive odor, insomnia, and fatigue. Six months prior to our initial consultation, he experienced four unexplained anxiety attacks and heart palpations. He was scared, felt he lost control of his health, and was willing to take on the nutritional and lifestyle changes necessary to be balanced and healthy. He could only afford two functional tests: the delayed food allergy test and the stool analysis test. The results were not surprising to me: sensitivity to eggs and dairy with the presence of candida albicans and clostridia in higher volumes. He also had high levels of Zonulin.

We removed dairy and eggs from his diet as well as wheat, oat, rye, and barley. Once on a low glycemic diet higher in proteins and vegetables along with an adjusted antifungal diet, herbs, and food supplements (such as pre-biotics and pro-biotics), he was able to reduce inflammation markers. Also, it increased metabolism speed, improved insulin resistance, improved digestion, improved gut flora, and balanced moodiness. Tim suffered only one anxiety attack over 8 months. In addition to that, he experienced no more heart palpations and lost 30 pounds!

No doubt, once Tim's gut bacteria replenished, his digestion system improved as his health condition shifted. Inflammation markers came down, nutrient deficiency gaps closed, and brain functionality improved while his weight became balanced.

Nutrition has the most powerful influence on our gut microbial activity. Food rich with friendly and beneficial bacteria such as bifidobacteria and lactobacillus found in yogurt, kefir, pre-biotic or pro-biotics, and fermented foods such as pickles, sauerkraut, kimchi, and miso can be very supportive to healthy gut micro-biome, fat digestion, and fat burning. If you are sensitive or allergic to dairy products, though, you should always avoid them!

As you can see, the secret is out. There is a direct correlation between your overall gut health and your ability to maintain a balanced weight! However, because the human digestive system is so complex, it is impossible to pinpoint your areas of concern, deficiencies, or any possible disorders on your own! I can't say this enough: Your health is too valuable to play guessing games with! Qualified nutritionists like me are here to help you find your balance, and we're more than happy to share in your joy with you when you see results!

THE SLEEP CONNECTION
TO WEIGHT GAIN

DOES SLEEP AFFECT YOUR WEIGHT?

Getting enough sleep is necessary to live a balanced life, yet 85% of my clients report feeling short on sleep! At the beginning of a consultation, most of my clients report waking up once every 2-3 hours during the night at least three nights a week. Whether they need to go to the bathroom, drink water, or they simply cannot sleep, it interferes with their sleep cycle and sleep quality, which can affect energy levels, leading to weight gain.

There are primarily three sub-groups of individuals who present more sleep deprivation patterns thus resulting in gaining weight due to a shortened cycle of sleep. These three sub-groups of individuals are pre-menopausal, menopausal for men and women, and young parents (moms in particular).

Sleep deprivation (getting very little sleep and/or circadian rhythms interrupted), affects your sleep quality which in turn will affect your metabolism. Gaining weight or an inability to lose weight in many cases is directly linked to sleep deprivation. There needs to be more awareness, understanding, and examination of this subject to find the best solutions!

WHY IS SLEEP A KEY COMPONENT IN YOUR WEIGHT LOSS JOURNEY?

Quality sleep restores the body's ability to regulate different metabolic functions which can affect your weight management. In the long run, gaining weight leads to an increased risk for heart disease, high insulin levels, and even diabetes.

Lack of sleep is related to increased hunger or appetite which affects the regulation of the peptides ghrelin and leptin. These hormones are responsible for signaling hunger and satisfaction to the brain. Lack of sleep will also increase your cravings for sweet or salty foods, thus affecting your blood sugar levels. Over time, this can lead to becoming overweight or even obese. These two hormones are the main reason why it's so hard to resist different high sugar snacks or caffeine when you feel sleep deprived. What ultimately happens is we trick ourselves into feeling like they are a fast energy booster.

Going for five hours or less without sleep affects hormonal changes. Consequently, it causes obesity, diabetes as well as other health problems. Problems such as: reduced insulin sensitivity (the hormone which controls blood sugar), increased inflammation, decreased fat oxidation, **cortisol** production (the hormone which regulates stress levels), reduced **thyroid** functionality (the hormone which regulates metabolism of every cell in the body). Also, it affects **serotonin** levels (affecting digestion, mood, behavior, memory, sleep and sexual functionality). All of these factors combined contribute to gaining weight. In fact, studies show that individuals who sleep 8½ hours burn twice as much fat as individuals who sleep five hours or less. Not to mention, those who got more sleep lost 10 pounds more than the second group over the course of 12 months![5]

Jeff is a 53-year-old diabetic who arrived at my office weighing 274 pounds. He is a construction worker and did physical work for most of his life, yet he had low energy levels and took medication to control his high cholesterol and blood sugar levels.

I quickly discovered that Jeff woke up every 90 minutes, every single night. He was incredibly sleep deprived! He learned how to live like this and just accepted it as an unchangeable aspect of his life. However, his health was detrimentally affected by his lack of sleep. On top of all that, his high cholesterol and blood sugar levels were getting worse, as were his memory and energy levels. He was apparently gaining weight, too – he'd gained 30 pounds just in the past year.

Once we started the program, our goal was to balance his body by reducing cholesterol levels and blood sugars while losing weight. He adapted to the nutritional program that was customized to his body's needs. He also made some lifestyle changes. He took control of his blood sugar and cholesterol levels while his weight began to drop. His sleep was prolonged to two hours, some nights even three hours until, eventually, after eight months in the program, he was able to sleep a full night and now he feels rejuvenated!

Jeff's weight was dropping and he was making tremendous progress. When Jeff finished the program, he weighed a svelte 190 pounds! He still maintains that weight today, even (as I'm writing this) 20 months after we finished his program! We were able to balance his blood sugar and cholesterol levels, too. He was happier and full of energy. He even returned to his long-lost hobby of fishing, so now I get fresh fish delivered to my doorstep whenever Jeff goes fishing. I feel so proud that I was part of Jeff's journey to improving his sleep and losing weight. He is just one of many whose lives have changed for the better after going through my program. Everybody can experience this same kind of change! There's no doubt about it: An adequate amount of sleep is a major factor in losing weight and maintaining a normal body weight.

WHY QUALITY OF SLEEP MATTERS

Many studies agree that a short sleep cycle is considered to be 6 hours or less. [1] Normal sleep also follows a certain pattern which allows regaining full bodily functionality the next day. In this sleeping pattern, Altering Rapid Eye Movement (REM) occurs during stage R. There is also non-REM sleep (NREM) which is repeated every 90 minutes. It is estimated that an average person spends 75% of their sleep time in NREM and about 25% in REM. Every sleep cycle begins with NREM stages of sleep which can extend into a stage known as "N3." During the first "N1" and "N2" stages, brain waves become slower and a person becomes disengaged from their surroundings. The "N3" stage is the deepest and the most restorative stage of sleep. It is during this stage when a decrease in heart rate, blood pressure, breathing, and muscle tension occurs. This allows energy to be restored. Later on in the sleep cycle, there are periods of REM sleep where the eyes dart back and forth. This is the part where dreaming happens as the brain becomes active again. [15] The length of each stage and overall sleep length can be influenced by various factors (daylight hours, meal times, alcohol consumption, temperature, exercising, and melatonin, gamma-aminobutyric acid (GABA), progesterone hormones). These hormones regulate and help to control sleep/wake cycles. It is important to know that excessive sleeping (for more than 10 hours) has been linked to weight gain as well. Sleeping cycles for people still differ, but the connection with weight gain is undeniable.

The hormones help to control sleep/wake cycles. Additionally, the natural body's circadian rhythm (biological clock) and the basic physiological need for sleep. It is important to know excessive sleeping for more than 10 hours has been linked to weight gain as well. Sleeping cycles for people still differ, but the connection with weight gain is undeniable.

WHAT CAN YOU DO TO IMPROVE YOUR QUALITY OF SLEEP?

It is possible to get healthy amounts of sleep and be in control of your body weight. If you do have melatonin hormone depletion, here are some suggestions that might improve your quality of sleep:

- **Avoid caffeine, at least in the afternoon.** This substance has a tendency to keep people in lighter stages of sleep which is much closer to a poor sleep stage. The best course of action would be to quit any caffeinated drink after 2 p.m. and switch to some kind of a decaf drink. It might be difficult at first to those who are used to this habit. The dependency urges people to think it gives them more energy, but it is only a temporary solution which does not provide efficient results. In most cases, people achieve much less with longer working hours than the ones who choose to sleep more.

- **Exercise** in moderation can increase human growth hormones, which has a positive effect of blunting cortisol and increasing the repair of your body. Exercising just before going to the bed can disturb your ability to fall asleep.

- **"TV Snacks"** - Keep track of your **eating habits!** It is especially important before going to sleep. Some people have a tendency to eat heavy meals and/or greasy foods such as pizza, potato chips, or popcorn while watching TV just before going to bed. If you're combining those snacks with beer or wine, then you're really creating a recipe for disaster. In fact, any kind of meal, big or small, is not a good idea before bed. This can cause trouble sleeping as well as problems with digestion and heartburn. These are just some of the reasons why so many studies and specialists do not suggest eating after 9 p.m. and especially not after midnight! You could start by trying lighter meals or healthy "TV snacks" to improve your sleep cycle.

- **Create routine** - Go to bed at the same time each night.
- **Avoid caffeine, alcohol, or nicotine** before bedtime, as these stimulants will prevent you from falling asleep or staying asleep for a sustained period of time.
- If you think your sleep deprivation might be related to **job stress or a busy schedule,** create a list of things you need to do the next day so you do not need to keep them in mind. Relax instead while trying to fall asleep.
- If necessary, supplement the above solutions with **melatonin** which can support your sleeping rhythm. . The suggested dose is 1-3 ml taken 60 to 90 minutes before bedtime. If you choose to take a melatonin supplement, please consult with your practitioner because quality of products and quantity do matter! **DO NOT MAKE THIS DECISION BY YOURSELF!**
- If necessary, consult with a **sleep specialist** who can provide further examination.

Getting a sufficient amount of sleep is critical for healthy and balanced metabolic pathways which support a balanced weight. Let's discuss how your hormones are connected to your weight gain or loss. [*1-16]

THE HORMONAL CONNECTION TO WEIGHT GAIN

Hormones play a key role when it comes to regulating your weight. If you have struggled to lose weight or to keep it off for more than 3 months, there is a very good chance you have hormonal imbalances. Hormones regulate and control every element of weight loss, including your metabolism, fat storage, appetite, and food cravings. Any hormone imbalances will challenge your goals to lose weight, regardless of the effort you put into it.

Meet Kim, a 38-year-old mom and full time employee who started my Balance Diet program hoping to lose 15 pounds. In our initial evaluation, she reported gaining extra weight over the last 12 months. She was fatigued, stressed, barely sleeping, skipping meals to catch up at work and yet somehow she felt hungry. Her memory declined to the point where she worried about being laid off from work. This was not an option for her or her family given the high cost of living in Silicon Valley, California. She was even complying with and following the diet more than many of my other clients. However, her weight did not change while the levels of frustration and disappointment were accumulating.

I suggested she take a comprehensive blood analysis, saliva hormone level and food sensitivity test. The results from those tests confirmed my suspicions. Her sugar levels were in the high range but still within the norm (Glucose 95). On top of that, HA1c levels were high (5.9), Triglycerides were on the high side (175), thyroid markers were completely out of range (TSH 4.5; T3 420; TPO antibody 67), and her cortisol levels (42 in the morning, 0.75 at night) respectively. She showed signs of low progesterone-estradiol ratio (34.5 which is consistent with estrogen dominance). The results also showed a gluten and casein (protein in dairy) sensitivity.

By addressing the underlying root cause of her stressors (food sensitivity, blood sugar regulation, thyroid function support, and inflammation reduction), we were able to help her achieve her goal. Once balanced both nutritionally and hormonally, she was able to see the desired changes to her weight, not to mention her energy, sleep, and memory all improved dramatically.

In 90% of my clinical experiences, I have found unexplained weight gain to be associated with hormonal imbalances. Hormones play a vital role when it comes to regulating weight, metabolism, blood sugar, and fat storage. Kim's example proves if you are not hormonally balanced, your weight will not come down regardless of your efforts.

WHAT ARE COMMON SYMPTOMS OF HORMONAL IMBALANCES?

Unexplained weight gain is one of the first symptoms of a hormonal imbalance. Other symptoms associated with hormonal imbalances are belly fat, fatigue, burnout, sluggishness, insomnia, decreased libido, sugar cravings, less lean muscle, no appetite or cravings, high body fat percentage, emotional eating, and stress. Many of my clients come to me seeking help because they feel they have lost control of their weight. Proper nutrition, exercise, and sleep are not enough to lose weight. Balancing your hormones will ease the process of losing weight and help you keep it off for more than 12 months.

Your hormonal system is dependent upon the abilities of the liver and kidneys to remove excessive self-production of hormones and toxins. Detoxification and excretion of any excess hormones is crucial for healthy and balanced hormonal circulation. If ignored, hypersensitivity, inflammation, and toxicity can build up, which can lead to further complications.

To make it even more complicated, you need to have the right enzymes to bond with the hormones receptors. This process targets the specific site cells that require these hormones. Enzymes are completely dependent upon the food you eat and affect both the quality and quantities of food. You also have to factor in the ability of your gut to break down foods to produce nutrients for your nourishment. The science is there to back it up: Nutrient deficiencies will affect your endocrine circadian rhythm and scale weight.

CAN NUTRITION BALANCE YOUR HORMONES?

Hormones are entirely dependent upon your daily food intake. You have to remember that hormones are essential fatty acids, or chemical messengers that target phototherapeutic elements thus increasing the cellular ability to "listen" to the hormonal message. [2]

This very delicate system fluctuates throughout the day. The chemicals produced by the endocrine glands can either increase or decrease the "speed" of the body's chemical reactions. These reactions regulate the nervous system and make them available through **organic nutrients and mineral ion concentration**. [1] The endocrine system is the most important system regulating your body's communication. It affects the brain, gut, immune system, heart, blood vessels, and more.

Nutrient deficiencies will put more stress on the endocrine system. Under chronic stress, B-vitamin levels begin to deplete. However, do you know anyone who is not stressed out these days? Personally, I don't.

A high carbohydrate diet demands an increase of the hormone insulin. In response to the changes of the sugar levels, the adrenal gland will produce more adrenaline as well as cortisol. These will circulate more of the thyroid hormones estrogen and testosterone.

Having overly high levels of **thyroid hormones** depletes vitamins A, C, and E as well as iodine, zinc, and selenium. Moreover, having overly high levels of **cortisol** will deplete vitamin B, amino acids, minerals, and iron.

High **insulin** levels deplete minerals, amino acids, and fatty acids. Elevated levels of blood sugar will create insulin resistance. Insulin resistance is a condition where cells resist the natural and healthy way of using insulin to transport glucose into the cell for energy production, ending up with extra insulin and internal inflammation.

High levels of stress can lead to high blood sugar, insulin resistance, and fat storage. Consuming a diet high in sugar, simple carbohydrates, or foods with a high glycemic index will prolong and enable this negative process, leading to metabolic syndrome (**high blood sugar, high blood pressure, high cholesterol, Polycystic Ovary Syndrome (PCOS), and type 2 diabetes**). All of these conditions are associated with increased inflammatory and cardiovascular markers. This is another reason why it is so important to speak with your nutritionist about what is happening inside your body if you want to regain control over your health and weight.

Changing your diet and nourishing your body's cells with the proper food is the key to balancing insulin resistance and weight loss. However, this is not always the only answer to weight gain.

Imbalances within sex hormones that decline with age, such as estrogen or testosterone, can also explain the challenges of balancing glucose levels, insulin resistance, and weight loss. Estrogen will lower insulin levels in women while testosterone will lower blood sugar in men. However, high levels of progesterone can raise blood sugar in women. Stress can contribute to the elevation of insulin levels by decreasing estrogen and testosterone levels. The same applies to excessive progesterone and DHEA.
[*1,2,4,5]

These examples are here to prove that **hormones are completely dependent upon our daily food intake.** Clearly, the hormonal circadian needs to come to a balancing point along with nutritional support before you will see any significant weight loss.

Nutrients play a key role in regulating cell and hormonal functions. Any changes within your food intake will affect this delicate balance. Balanced hormones require a balanced diet that can lead to a healthy weight.

ENVIRONMENTAL TOXINS AFFECTING YOUR HORMONES

Environmental toxins such as pesticides, DDT, herbicides, and fungicides are interfering with your endocrine system regulation. So are pollution from plastic bottles, metal or aluminum food cans, toys, cosmetics, and detergents. Chemicals such as Phthalates (industrial compounds known technically as dialkyl or alkyl aryl esters of 1,2-benzenedicarboxylic acid), PBBs (Polybrominated Biphenyls) or Bisphenol A (BPA) are all interfering with your endocrine system regulation, leading to weight gain.

Obesity Reviews published a paper titled "Energy Balance and Pollution by Organochlorines and Polychlorinated Biphenyls" in 2003. This article outlines the effects toxins have on the metabolic rate and weight regulation via various mechanisms. The authors conclude that pesticides and PCBs (from industrial pollution) released from fat tissue during weight loss lower the metabolic rate. The authors go on to conclude that we should lose a little weight to reduce the risk of cardiovascular and degenerative diseases, but not too much because we could poison our metabolism. [3]

Studies document that when individuals change their nutrition from non-organic to organic food, the levels of pesticides in the body decrease. [4] Likewise, avoiding canned food reduces bisphenol A levels. [5]

One of my recent clients, Jean, a 37 year-old female diagnosed with a hyperthyroid condition. Her main symptoms were chronic fatigue, diarrhea, heat intolerance, sweating, irritability, moodiness, and weight gain. Literally speaking, her thyroid was not functioning properly. We tested her using the Toxic Organic chemical test, which came back with high levels of several chemicals. Among them were **Phthalates,** commonly found in after shave lotions, aspirin, cosmetics, detergents, foods microwaved with plastic covers, oral pharmaceutical drugs, plastic bags, hair sprays, nail polish, nail polish remover, and skin care products. Removing phthalates compounds (as much as possible) from her immediate environment while supporting her nutritionally reduced many of her body's symptoms to the point where she could modify her medication dosages and even lose weight.

Yes, environmental toxins are part of life and we most likely will not be able to get rid of them completely until making further policy changes. However, we can make better choices by reducing our exposure to chemicals. When we choose to eat organic foods, the body has less stress and does not collapse, as you can see from Jean's experience.

Hormones balance each other to create homeostasis. This is so important that even if one hormone is not balanced it creates hormonal dysfunction. Stress, nutrient deficiencies, sleep, sugar levels, inflammation, toxicity, and age are some of the many factors which influence this delicate hormonal circadian rhythm which can contribute to weight gain.

WHAT HOMONES CAUSE WEIGHT GAIN?

The seven major hormones I see within each of my clients are:

- Adrenal-Cortisol levels (stress)
- Sugar levels - Insulin, Leptin, Glucose and Hemoglobin A1C (energy)
- Sex hormone levels - Testosterone, DHEAS, Estradiol, Progesterone, IGF-1 (growth hormone)
- Thyroid levels - TSH (Thyroid Stimulating Hormone), Free T3, Free T4, Reverse T3 (energy)
- Vitamin D levels
- Melatonin levels (sleep)
- The Leptin and Ghrelin Hormones

THE ADRENAL-CORTISOL-DHEA CONNECTION TO YOUR WEIGHT GAIN

Cortisol is an essential hormone for a balanced body. It is a steroid hormone produced by the adrenal glands along with DHEA. The hormones cortisol and DHEA are involved in your body's development, growth, immune response, stress, modulation of the thyroid, regulating blood sugars, blood pressure, and cardiovascular function. More interesting than that is how cortisol plays a key role within regulating energy by "picking" carbohydrates (glycogen into glucose) as well as fats and proteins (catabolism) to support the metabolism of these elements.

Cortisol is also known as the "fight or flight" hormone. When stress increases, cortisol levels will rise to meet the challenge. Unfortunately, modern life keeps us on "fight or flight" mode until the adrenals reach their exhaustion point. Weight gain will be one of the first symptoms you notice if this happens.

Adrenals also regulate the metabolism of blood sugars to fuel the body's energy. When you're over stressed, cortisol gets off balance as blood sugars and insulin levels increase, thus creating insulin resistance. Consequently, appetite will increase, sleep interruptions will occur, energy production declines, moodiness, fatigue, cravings for junk foods, and over consumption of coffee or sodas will occur. This leads to the body building up visceral fat storage as a survival method. The fat storage is mainly around the waist, which of course leads to weight gain! [*1,2,3,4,5,6]

Cortisol also transports triglycerides from storage to the visceral fat cells and then into the adipocytes cells. These develop into mature fat cells and are negative contributors to weight gain. The more unresolved chronic stress (mental, emotional, or physical) you have, the more fat storage is happening. [*1,2,3,4,5,6]

On top of that, if you are in your midlife years, there are other factors to consider such as hormone production naturally declining as well as the adrenal glands taking over hormone production. They do this in an attempt to meet your hormonal needs because the body senses something is missing. The result is an increased demand on the adrenal glands, which leads to cortisol over production. This means more fat storage, excessive blood sugars within abdominal fat cells as a fuel source, and, at the same time, retention of these fats until stress levels declines. Therefore, you end up with weight gain without the ability to reduce these extra pounds, regardless of your efforts. You have to support your adrenals nutritionally; otherwise, more tissue damage and inflammation occur. This weakens the immune system and lowers the retention of sodium ions. Over time, this leads to reduction or the stomach's ability to manage acids, which may trigger conditions such as **gastritis or ulcers.**

Saliva tests can measure your cortisol levels and indicate if there is adrenal dysfunction or adrenal fatigue. Healthy and properly functioning adrenals are vital for vibrant health. Without them, there is no way to make necessary changes to weight.

HOW IS INSULIN RESISTANCE CONNECTED WITH WEIGHT GAIN?

The hormone insulin was discussed earlier in this book. High levels of blood sugar create insulin resistance which can be measured by elevated fasting blood sugar levels.

Insulin resistance is a condition where the body cannot absorb glucose into its cells properly or efficiently. If you will, it is a condition where your body has a weak response to the hormone insulin. Insulin controls the glucose amount in cells that will be used immediately. The presence of insulin indicates "a fed state," which facilitates the production of glycogen (stored glucose) in the liver and muscle as well as triglycerides in adipose cells. It is clear, that the storage of glycogen is limited. It is around 500g (depending on the muscle mass). Excess glucose is later stored as triglycerides. Insulin also causes fat and prevents the breakdown of it. [*1,2,3]

In those with insulin resistance condition, the cells resist the natural and healthy way of using insulin to transport glucose into the cells for energy production. Your body tries to create extra insulin as an attempt to help glucose enter the cells, but what really happens is internal inflammation. Other potential contributors to insulin resistance are chronic stress, high-glycemic load diet (gluten or gluten-free), smoking, lack of exercise, and toxins.

To be able to lose weight, it is crucial to control insulin and avoid insulin resistance, which can lead to diabetes if not balanced. [*4,5]

Remember as I told you earlier in the book: Higher levels of stress lead to high blood sugar, thus creating insulin resistance and increasing fat storage. This is exactly why it is so important to nourish your body with the proper diet customized for you individually. Changing your diet will help you balance insulin resistance and will lead to weight loss.

Another potential factor I mentioned earlier is an imbalance of sex hormones. Again, even though they decline with age, estrogen and testosterone play a major role in balancing your weight, as do insulin levels. Estrogen will lower insulin levels in women while testosterone will lower blood sugar in men. However, high levels of progesterone can raise blood sugar in women. Also, stress can contribute to the elevation of insulin levels by decreasing estrogen and testosterone levels. The same can be said for excessive progesterone and DHEA.

The bottom line is that there needs to be a balancing point within your hormonal circadian rhythm. The right solution here is doing it through nutritional support so you can benefit from potential significant weight loss.

THE SEX HORMONE CONNECTION TO WEIGHT GAIN

The three sex hormones I am most often looking at when weight loss is slowed down or not as expected regardless of the nutritional or exercise efforts are **estrogen, progesterone,** and **testosterone**. To simplify this complex network of hormonal communication, I decided to put it in bullet points for you:

Some Facts:

1. Fluctuating hormones such as estrogen, testosterone and progesterone impact your **appetite, metabolism, and fat storage.**

2. **Estrogen** is involved in almost 400 bodily functions. Among them are increased metabolic rate, improved insulin sensitivity, regulation of body temperature, improved sleep, improved blood flow, and increased magnesium uptake and utilization. In addition, estrogen helps in memory support and bone health, and supports the neurotransmitter serotonin that decreases depression, irritability, anxiety, and pain sensitivity.

3. **Progesterone** promotes regular sleep patterns, prevents bloating, maintains libido, fosters a calming effect on the body, stimulates bone building, and thickens the uterine lining to promote survival of a fertilized egg (ovum).

4. **Estrogen and progesterone** synchronize and complement each other to achieve optimum balance. We need both hormones, but in the right ratio.

5. **Estrogen** is produced within **fat cells.** Our body works harder to convert calories from food into fat to increase levels of estrogen, which increases weight gain. In simple words – **the more weight your body carries, the more estrogen you produce.**

6. **High Levels of Estrogen** - Leads to a condition known as estrogen dominance. This occurs when estrogen levels are deficient, normal, or excessive while progesterone is too low to balance the estrogen levels.

7. **Progesterone** levels are declining even before menopause. When progesterone levels are low, estrogen levels are high.

8. Stress, antidepressants, excessive use of arginine, high blood sugar, and hypothyroidism can lead to **low levels of progesterone.**

9. A drop-in **estrogen** can increase the appetite while decreasing the metabolism, which affects **weight gain.**

10. Hot flashes and night sweats are not the only symptoms men and women will experience when the balance between **estrogen and progesterone** is off. Other major symptoms of **excessive estrogen** include **weight gain (up to 20 pounds),** migraine headaches, poor sleep, poor memory, foggy thinking, moodiness, depression, anxiety, panic attacks, swollen breasts, heavy periods, hypothyroidism, autoimmune disease, uterine fibroids, bloating, gas, indigestion, bone loss, pain in the ankles,

knees, wrists, shoulders, and heels, as well as cold hands and feet.

11. **Estrogen** recycling and metabolism is dependent on a **healthy gut.**

12. Excessive **cortisol and estrogen** will inhibit <u>thyroid functionality</u>. Those hormones need to work in synchronicity with each other. The estrogen will inhibit the conversion of T4 to T3 leading to a sluggish metabolism which will affect your weight.

13. **Insulin resistance** will decline with the production of 17-Hydrox-pregnenolone activity, which leads to an increase of <u>SHBG</u> (Sex hormone-binding globulin), <u>DHEA-S</u> (Dehydroepiandrosterone-Sulfate), and testosterone. This also leads to higher free estrogen levels.

14. When **testosterone** levels are dropping, the body's **metabolism is slowing down.** As a result, fewer calories transform into lean muscle mass. This means higher risks for weight gain.

15. Healthy **testosterone** levels regulate body <u>fat metabolism</u>, support <u>lean muscles</u>, support the <u>metabolic rate</u>, <u>improve memory and bone</u> strength, and support production of the <u>neurotransmitter norepinephrine</u> in the brain.

16. **Aromatase** is an enzyme found in skin, fat, bone, and brain cells. Its purpose is to convert testosterone into estrogen.

17. Low levels of **testosterone** are a significant and independent risk factor for <u>metabolic syndrome</u> (high blood pressure, high levels of cholesterols, high blood sugar, insulin resistance, and weight gain).

18. Low **testosterone** and obesity reinforce each other, trapping men in a spiral of weight gain and hormonal imbalance.

19. **Testosterone** has beneficial effects on insulin regulation, lipid profiles, and blood pressure.

20. Declining **testosterone** levels cause a steady rise in C-reactive protein (CRP), a marker of inflammation, which affects cholesterol levels, insulin resistance, and weight.

Hormone levels will affect weight gain. Hormones need to synchronize with each other in order for you to achieve a healthy weight. Weight loss involves more than just balancing the hormones. Making nutrition and lifestyle changes such as reducing excessive exercise, improving sleep, minimizing toxin exposure, and reducing stress are necessary in order to achieve a healthy weight. [*1-19]

THE THYROID CONNECTION TO WEIGHT GAIN

The thyroid is another critical gland that regulates **appetite, weight, and metabolism**. The thyroid gland is one part of a very complex hormonal system. Many people experience weight gain, weakness, sleep disturbances, hot flashes, low sex drive, low blood pressure, memory decline, depression, or mood swings during periods of unexplained weight gain, depending on thyroid levels.

An underactive thyroid is generally associated with some weight gain. Weight loss is common among individuals with hyperthyroidism. In most cases, the weight gain is due to an accumulation of salt and water and the average gain is 5-10 pounds.

When T3 levels drop, LDL cholesterol levels will rise due to a slower metabolism of fats. This leads to the depletion of essential fatty acids, which affects mitochondria energy production. As a result, glucose levels rise, and most likely insulin resistance will be developed. Weight gain will be the consequence from this chain of biological reactions. [*6]

Checking your thyroid functionality is necessary if you suspect imbalances. It is best to ask your physician to run a Comprehensive Thyroid Panel instead of checking checking your Thyroid Stimulating Hormone (TSH) levels by themselves. If you only check TSH levels, there will be some challenges when it comes to early detection of any possible complications. TSH levels will not necessarily be elevated at the early stage of a declining thyroid gland. If your doctor measures only the TSH levels, they may seem in the normal range. However, you may still show symptoms of something being off: fatigue, becoming overweight, cravings for sweets or salt, restlessness, and moodiness.

A Comprehensive Thyroid Panel includes the following biomarkers, which provide a greater picture of your overall thyroid function and unexplained weight changes:

- **Thyroid-Stimulating Hormone (TSH)** - Evaluates overall thyroid function
- **Total Thyroxine (T4)** - Measures the total amount of T4 produced by the thyroid gland
- **Free Thyroxine (T4)** - Measures the amount of T4 available to the cells and tissues
- **Free Tri-iodothyronine (T3)** - Measures the amount of T3 (the active form of the hormone) available to the cells and tissues
- **Reverse T3** - Measures the non-functioning form of the active hormone T3
- **Antithyroglobulin Antibody (ATA)** - Often measured along with TPO, these antibodies can attack the proteins involved in the production of thyroid hormones, thus rendering them dysfunctional
- **Thyroid Peroxidase Antibody (TPO)** - Often measured along with ATA, these antibodies can

attack proteins involved in the production of thyroid
hormones, thus rendering them dysfunctional

The Thyroid gland is not an isolated organ; **it is part of the
hormonal system**. It is counter-dependent on the total healthy
hormonal sum. It is for this reason that the thyroid gland requires
a holistic examination.

There are other factors and questions to answer outside of
the thyroid gland when it comes to weight loss. For example, how
well is the liver functioning to detoxify? How healthy is your gut?
Do you experience diarrhea, heartburn, Irritable Bowel Syndrome
(IBS), acid reflux, or stomach aches? How strong is your immune
system? Are you sensitive or allergic to any foods? Do you have
any other diagnosis of autoimmune diseases?

Like any other hormones, T4 and T3 can be affected by
nutrient deficiencies. Nutrient deficiencies can decrease self-
production of T4 and T3 as well as the conversion of T4 to T3. For
example, what are your levels of vitamin B12, D, A, Iodine, and
Iron [2,3,4]? How is your overall hormonal functionality (adrenal,
insulin, vitamin D, etc.)? Have you been exposed to environmental
toxins? Have you been exposed to biological toxins such as
bacteria, yeast, or parasites? What are your stress levels like? Are
you taking medications such as beta-blockers, birth control pills,
estrogen replacements, lithium, phenytoin, or theophylline? All of
those medications prevent the conversion of T4 to T3. [4,5] Have you
undergone chemotherapy treatment? Are you taking supplements
and if so, what kind? How well are you sleeping? Do you exercise
regularly? These all factor into the greater picture of your overall
health and well-being.

The truth is that healthy thyroid regulation needs to be
balanced to optimize health and healthy weight.

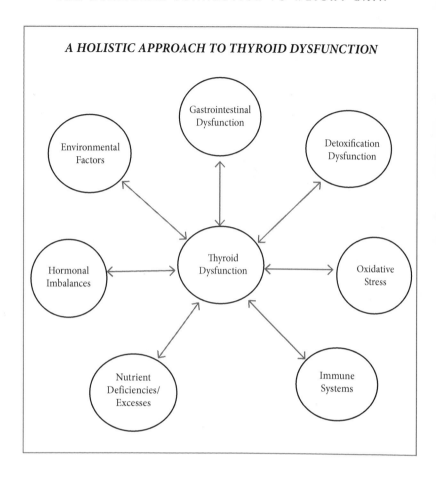

A HOLISTIC APPROACH TO THYROID DYSFUNCTION

THE LEPTIN AND GHRELIN CONNECTION TO WEIGHT GAIN

Another set of key hormones that influence weight gain are **Ghrelin and Leptin**. These two hormones regulate hunger and feelings of satisfaction. Most of my clients do not feel hungry when they start the program. They can go up to 6 or even 8 hours without any food. Others will claim they are so busy they only have time for one meal a day.

Leptin is a hormone secreted by fat cells. It sends a signal to the brain when we have enough energy stored to suppress the appetite. [1] This means eating less food, which creates a negative cycle of starvation, ending with weight gain. [2]

Levels of Leptin will decline naturally with age, which also affects weight. Healthy fats can boost levels of Leptin if you consume foods containing Eicosapentaenoic acid (EPA). Fish such as sardines and salmon contain EPA. Getting enough sleep is also imperative because lack of sleep negatively affects Leptin hormones while increasing Ghrelin. [7] Perhaps even more impressive is the fact that high levels of insulin, as discussed earlier, prevent the Leptin signal from creating more energy storage in the body as glycogen or fat.

Insulin is the hormone that tells the cells to pick up glucose from the bloodstream. It is also the major energy storage hormone in the body. It signals cells to store energy, as either glycogen or fat. [5] This is one more reason why weight gain occurs if there is not balance in your diet.

Ghrelin is the hormone that regulates hunger levels. This means high levels of Ghrelin create uncontrolled cravings. Ghrelin works directly with the hunger center of the brain. It activates the brain's reward response to highly addictive sweet, salty, and fatty foods. This uncontrolled hunger gets even worse after dinner, before bedtime, when you're tired or when you're watching TV. The result is always the same: weight gain. [4,6]

From other studies, it is evident that diets high in healthy proteins such as chicken, turkey, lamb, whole cheese, or omega-3 eggs (as long as you are not sensitive to them) combined with adequate sleep could support decreasing your levels of Ghrelin. [3] Over time, this will help you balance your weight.

Hormones are dependent on organic nutrient and mineral ion concentration, if you are nutritionally depleted, it will affect your hormones regulation. Moreover, hormones need to synchronize with each other in order for the body to achieve healthy weight

You should test your hormone levels before taking any intervention steps. You cannot afford to guess when it comes to health and well-being. After testing, developing a nutritional plan based on the results will restore your balance. In most cases, it is a simple saliva test to measure your body's "free" hormone levels, which are the **active** hormones available for use by tissues. This provides an accurate reading of unbound hormone levels in circulation (5%). **Don't guess, test!**

Nutritionally, you want to minimize sugars, carbohydrates, and caffeine. Limit xenoestrogen exposure. *Eat green, colorful, phyto-chemically dense, local, non-GMO foods and as little processed food as possible.*

Use **ONLY** high quality supplements that can support this delicate hormonal balance. Support your gut, liver detoxification, and the two other major hormone glands: adrenal and thyroid. Exercise in moderation and drink plenty of water and herbal teas to stay hydrated and nourished.

Again, hormone imbalances in men and women absolutely affect weight. This very complex network of hormonal messages requires nutrition and lifestyle changes such as reducing excessive exercise, improving sleep, minimizing toxin exposure, and reducing stress first, before experiencing weight loss, regardless if your diet is gluten or gluten free.

THE BALANCED DIET

If you have reached this part of the book, then you have discovered the reason why you can't lose weight and keep it off. Basically, it is because of one or more of your body systems that is off balance. Also, I'm sure you realize there are many reasons why your body held onto weight, despite the diets or workout routine you are using. There's a lot more that goes into the process of losing weight. It is clear that the "calorie in, calorie out" myth is untrue. It is more of the overall systemic balance that needs to be achieved while reducing weight. It involves the six body systems that are crucial to achieving and maintaining a balance for optimum weight that reflects as optimum health. Presented in these body systems are nutrients availability, energy production, gut efficiency, hormone levels, food sensitivity, and healthy immune system. Sleep, stress, genetics, toxicity (biological and environmental), and liver detoxification are all key factors in the weight-loss equation, making it unique experience for every person.

The Balance Diet was designed to reach the balance point of each of the six body systems simultaneously, especially if one or more systems are unbalanced. If so, they create more stress on your body and therefore, weight loss cannot be achieved. It is a holistic system-oriented approach that transforms one's eating habits with **whole, dense, diverse, and organic food**. For some individuals, the Balanced Diet will bring not just nutritional changes but lifestyle changes as well.

Taking good care of your health requires functional tests along with conventional tests to address the underlying causes of your body's imbalances that are presented as your body's symptoms like weight gain. Tests like food sensitivity, nutritional status, digestive function, hormone levels, and biological and environmental toxins are part of the functional tests offered in my clinic. **There is not a one-size-fits-all nutritional plan.** Every one of us has a unique biochemistry that needs to be measured so you can achieve optimum health and lose weight. If you connect with me, a **Personalized Nutritional Program** will be designed based on the data collected so you can reach your balanced point. It is a preventive care rather than the acute and emergency care that is deeply entrenched in conventional medicine. The goal is to optimize the biological functioning in our body's core physiological systems.

"OPTIMAL" CHANGE WITH BALANCE

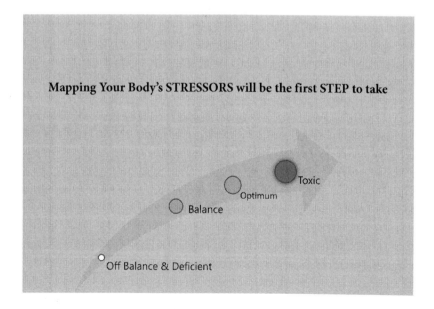

Mapping Your Body's STRESSORS will be the first STEP to take

Toxic

Optimum

Balance

Off Balance & Deficient

According to the U.S. Centers for Disease Control and Prevention (CDC), it is evident that over 74% of all adult men and 64% of all adult women are overweight. This means that almost 70% of the population is at a significant risk of chronic disease and illnesses that hold them back from losing weight. Nonetheless, if only they could reach the balance point for their bodies, then they could easily achieve weight loss.

The results are amazing. The success rate on the Balance Diet is 85% to 95%, and it is measurable. For some, it will be a completely restored optimum function of the six body systems, while others could see significant improvements in their body symptoms. Blood markers will improve, nutrients, digestion, energy, immunity and hormones will be at the balance point, and weight will come down. As long as you continue to consume high quantities of quality nutrients, weight loss will occur and can be maintained.

> **Maintaining** the "new" weight achieved depends on quality and high quantities of the FOOD you consume daily.

PERSONALIZED NUTRITIONAL PLAN - START TO CARRY YOURSELF TO A BALANCE POINT

The good news is that you can start the Balance Diet as soon as you finish reading this chapter, even if you are not a client of Mor's Nutrition and More and you have not completed the functional tests. However, this part of the book includes ONLY general nutritional guidance and DOES NOT take into consideration the root causes of your unbalanced body systems for weight gain.

If you choose to adopt the Balance Diet without any functional nutritional tests, you might face some challenges along this nutritional journey. It is highly recommended that you run the tests to discover the root causes of your body's imbalances. In addition to nutrition and lifestyle changes, you may also need botanical medicines, nutritional supplements, a therapeutic nutritional plan, or detoxification programs.

LET'S GET STARTED!

Start by following these easy steps:

BODY HYDRATION

Go water – Most of my clients at the starting point are simply dehydrated. Either because they drink too many cups of coffee, sodas, bottles of flavored water, alcohol, a combination of all of the above. They are over stressed, sleep deprived, smoke, do not exercise, have low energy and experience brain fogginess. They are wired and tired. All are negative factors that keep you dehydrated.

Symptoms of water dehydration: Dry skin, dry mouth, bad breath, muscle cramps, headaches, thirst, constipation, minimal urine, dizziness or lightheadedness, sleepiness or tiredness, low blood pressure, irritability and confusion, and rapid heartbeat and breathing are some of your body signals for dehydration. You may also have **food cravings** especially for **sweets and carbs**, which **slows down your metabolism and fat burning.**

Water is necessary for all digestion and respiratory processes. Water will transport oxygen, nutrients, and bio-waste into and outside your cells and provide you with electrolytes like chloride, fluoride, magnesium, calcium, potassium, and sodium, all of which we need to function and balance our weight.

Yes, you want to drink half of your body weight in ounces on daily basis.

If your weight is 160 pounds, that means you need to drink at least 80 ounces of water every day. If you are working out, or if you are living in hot weather, then you want to drink much more water to replace the loss of fluids from sweating.

If you drink enough water, your urine color will be clear to light yellow. If you are taking food supplements, most likely the color of your urine will turn lighter and brighter. Darker yellow is an indication of less water, meaning you are dehydrated.

Obviously, you don't want to drink more than your body needs and develop "water intoxication." Moderation and balance, using your common sense, and considering other factors like weather, exercise, age, gender, and medications will lead to sustainable liquid intake.

Water does not have any caloric value as long as it's pure and clean. If you use flavored water, you are "earning" the additives, the flavors, and most likely the high corn fructose syrups, sucrose, and sweeteners which are all adding to your body's imbalance stressors which will support the negative mechanism of gaining weight. On the other hand, clean pure water, herbal teas, and soups will provide you with positive support for any weight loss program. [*3,13,16,34]

> Pure **water, herbal teas and soups** will provide you with positive support for any weight loss program.

WHAT ABOUT DRINKING COFFEE?

Many of my clients will drink coffee and mistakenly consider it as equal as water intake. However, the fact is that coffee is dehydrating us even more and depletes us of nutrients like B and C vitamins. It also consumes more minerals such as potassium, magnesium, zinc, and calcium. Coffee interrupts our sleep cycle by depleting melatonin production. It also increases anxiety levels by depleting serotonin production. Coffee can increase adrenal over production of the catecholamines hormones, epinephrine and norepinephrine the "flight-fight" hormones that our adrenals will release under stress. All of these issues are negative factors of coffee that will promote weight gain. Also, drinking 3-6 cups a day will increase insulin resistance, which increases fat storage, greater oxidation of fat, and risk for diabetic and cardiovascular disease. [1,20,41]

You may think that up to three cups of coffee a day is safe amount of caffeine. It might be the case later in the program, but not at the starting point where you need to bring your body to a balance point. Only after achieving balance point, you can drink 1-2 cups of coffee a day. In most cases, at this stage of the process, people will notice the adverse effects of drinking coffee. I find that cutting out coffee is the hardest step most individuals will face under the Balance Diet. Herbal teas (hot or at room temperature), fresh water with herbs like: mint, sage, lemon grass, or organic ginger and lemon, cold fermented kambucha, or a bowl of soup are good enough to help with the challenge of giving up coffee for 21 to 28 days. Eating raw fresh organic arugula leaves or grapefruit when in season can be added to reduce the need for caffeine.

> NO coffee for the first 3-6 weeks of the Balance Diet
> When adding back coffee, try to drink up to 2 cups a day

WHAT ABOUT DRINKING ALCOHOL?

At the starting point, you want to limit alcohol consumption altogether. I have nothing against one or two glasses (4 ounces each) of wine occasionally, for special occasions such as holidays parties etc. In fact, I like to have red wine occasionally too. The challenge is when you over consume it. Many of my youngest clients drink alcohol over the weekend. It is also challenging if you drink alcohol on daily basis. Studies show that moderate alcohol consumption (150ml of red wine) will support blood lipid profiles, decrease lethal blood clots, increase coronary blood flow, reduce blood pressure, improve insulin sensitivity, and support the immune system. [21] Drinking wine and beer in moderation after reaching the balance point, will contribute to your overall health. This is evident since it adds soluble fibers, minerals, vitamins, and polyphenols like resveratrol, which support the immune system, prevent cancer, and cool down inflammation with the polyphenol xanthohumol – an anti-inflammatory flavonoid that is found in beer and supports the immune system. [19] Most beers are brewed with a large proportion of wheat or malted barley. If you are sensitive or allergic to gluten, you want to avoid beer with no questions. Even the gluten free versions of beer are brewed from sorghum, buckwheat, millet, and brown rice which can be challenging for some of us.

Alcoholic beverages are high in calories. In one glass of red wine, there are about 80-120 calories. There are 250-400 calories if you drink one glass of beer, even if it's gluten-free. Do the math – if you drink 1-3 glasses of wine over one meal you are adding about 80-250 calories per one glass of drink on top of what you ate.

You should know that our bodies will break down alcohol at a rate of one drink (glass) per each hour. Be smart and monitor your alcohol consumption. Always eat before drinking alcohol to prevent it from affecting your blood sugar levels which can increase inflammation levels.

Drinking too much alcohol affects your nutrient concentrations in the long run. Studies show that alcohol inhibits fat absorption and therefore, absorption of vitamins A, E, and D will decline. Vitamins B1, B3, B5, B6, B9, B12, C, and zinc will also drop due to alcohol consumption. [14,19,21,42] Down the road, nutritional deficiencies will affect your overall health and cause several adverse effects to your brain, blood sugar, and skin as well as headaches, intestinal problems, fatigue, anemia, hormonal imbalances, estrogen metabolism, inflammation, and weight gain.

Keep in mind, coffee and alcohol act as diuretics which causes the kidneys to secret water but not toxins, which keeps and prolongs the viscous cycle of dehydration, nutrient deficiencies, toxicity, and weight gain.

> Over consumption of coffee or alcohol will keep you:
>
> **toxic, dehydrated, nutritionally depleted and overweight.**

DID YOU SAY VEGETABLES?

Eating vegetables is crucial for your health. Vegetables provide us with the phytonutrients we all need daily. If you do not eat enough vegetables, there is no other way your body can get those nutrients. Our body simply can't supply these nutrients. Phytonutrients, like carotenonids and flavonodis are critical towards maintaining a healthy immune system, alkaline our blood, protect against cancers, heart disease, high blood pressure, vision, macular degeneration, and weight loss.

Vegetables are a rich source of vitamins A, C, and K, and minerals like calcium, magnesium, folate, potassium, and iron. They are also rich in dietary fibers to improve and regulate our digestive system, and chlorophyll, a key alkaline component.

I cannot more clearly express the importance of eating vegetables every single day. You want to eat between **4-6 cups of vegetables a day**. At least 50% of the vegetables need to be green, dark leafy vegetables (a minimum of two cups a day). You want to diversify your options and eat all kinds of dark green leafy vegetables and not stick only to iceberg lettuce. **Vibrant and super powerful dark green vegetables help maintain a healthy and balanced body.** Such vegetables include: spinach, kale, Swiss chard, turnip greens, broccoli, collard greens, rapini, dandelion green, mustard greens, bok choy, red clovers and watercress. You can get the same nutritional value from dark green herbs like parsley, basil, dill, chives, cilantro, and green onions

You can use dark leafy vegetables and create fresh salads daily. You can add them to your juices, your soups, and your eggs. You can even steam them and cook with them, in addition to using them as a wrap with tuna salad, chicken salad, tofu, or avocado.

To meet the needed requirements, I have two rules that simply work:

a. **The 3 x 3 Rule:**

To increase your vegetable intake daily, salads are your best and easiest option. Think of a two-layer salad:

1. THE BASE - **a mix of 3 different types of dark leafy greens:** lettuce (any kind), kale, spinach, Swiss chard, etc. Any combination works.

2. THE TOP – add at least **3 different types of vegetables** to your base green salad. Vegetables like: carrots, cucumbers, radishes, celery, tomatoes, peas, cauliflower, broccoli, mushrooms, etc.

3. GO FRESH, **organic, local and seasonal.**

b. **The DRO Rule – Diversify, Rotate, and eat Organic:** Make sure you are diversifying, rotating, and eating organic foods as much as possible, especially with vegetables. Make it a daily habit. Eat different colors of vegetables. The pigment color is rich in phytonutrients, the foundation of health.

Many of my clients at the starting point will have 1 -2 salads over a period of 7 days. This method puts you automatically on a nutrient deficiency baseline, which takes a huge toll on your overall health. Simply add more vegetables to your daily intake.

Raw, cooked, steamed or baked are all good cooking methods that can support your health and your goal to lose weight.

We need to eat clean foods and in large quantities to reach the nutrient volume our body requires to maintain optimum and balanced health and stable weight. I find this is the challenge my clients struggle with the most. The concept of eating less food and therefore losing weight is passé. In fact, it will create more stress and will hold you back from losing weight. Besides, eating less food will deplete your nutrient levels and create more negative stressors on your body, such as inflammation, hormonal imbalance, and sleep interruption.

The 3 x 3 Salad Formula

You want to have 2 salads a day.

Salad Size: two times a cereal bowl size each (approx. 24 oz)

Salad Base: mix of 3 different dark green leafy vegetables

Additional Vegetables: at least 3 more different vegetables

Salad Dressing (optional): *2 tablespoons of oil, 1 tablespoon of apple cider vinegar, salt and pepper*

(note: look at our recipe section for more salad dressing options)

"SMART" CALORIES TO FUEL YOUR CELLS

You probably know a calorie is a measure of energy which fuels your body. All foods have calories and different foods have different amounts of calories. Calories are provided by carbohydrates, fats, and proteins. Without energy, our body would not function.

We need at least 1,000 to 1,400 calories per day to get enough energy to fuel our key organs and survive. This minimum number is called the Resting Metabolic Rate (RMR), which varies depends on age, gender, weight, and muscle mass. **However, this is not enough to keep our daily routine activity.** We need to add in 400 to 600 calories per day in order to meet the requirements of our body.

If you go over the number your body requires, you will gain weight. It takes an excess of 3,500 calories to to gain one pound (lb.) of fat. For example, if your body needs 1,800 calories a day to maintain your current weight, and you consume 2,300 calories a day, then by the end of the week you would gain one lb.

Obviously, in order to lose weight, you need to reduce the number of calories consumed. **The challenge is how to lose weight while staying healthy.** Proteins, fats, and vegetables are the key nutrients to fuel your cells with energy on a low calorie daily intake. The challenge here is what other foods you are adding to your vegetables and what method of preparation you are using.

Vegetables are low in calories, high in their phytonutrients and water content. I call it a **"smart" calorie.** This is not the only factor you want to look at.

Many people add vegetables to their diet when they are ready to shed some weight. Barbara was one of many of my clients that chose to increase her daily vegetable intake to lose weight. She added salads and some baked or steamed vegetables. She also snacked on carrots and snow peas with hummus on a regular basis. Her weight "stuck" on 186 pounds for almost 8 months. Her cholesterol levels were high (total cholesterol 263) regardless of the effort she made. She was confused and frustrated when she reached my clinic. Evaluating her food intake, it seemed that she was using ¼ cup of shredded cheese with each salad, which added about 110 calories to her meal, and two servings of commercial ranch salad dressing, which added about 250 more calories (on average one serving of ranch salad dressing is about 145 calories). True, she was eating salad every day, though she added about 360 calories that were high in fat and high in sugar. In fact, that did not just slow her metabolism, but it also increased her cholesterol level risking her heart and blocking her ability to lose weight. Taking off the shredded cheese and replacing the commercial ranch salad dressing with a homemade delicious and nutritious salad dressing did what was close to magic for her. After ten weeks, she lost 15 pounds. Her cholesterol levels went down to a normal range after a few more weeks. As far as I know, she still balances.

Not every calorie is equal. Eat smart!

Moderation is the key to success, along with moderate exercise. You will be able to achieve your goal and maintain healthy weight for a long period of time. Smart calories support you more than you think, so making better food choices will support your health for a longer period of time.

> Eat vegetable as much as you can!
> For successful RESULTS eat a minimum of two cups a day
> Nutrient DENSE, dietary FIBERS, low CALORIES

STARCHY VEGETABLES

Starchy vegetables are sub groups of the vegetables family. **Potatoes, corn, pumpkins, sweet potatoes, yams, beets, jicama, parsnips, taro root, carrots, acorn squash, and butternut squash** are part of this family.

Starchy vegetables are a great source of vitamins A and C, beta-carotene, lutein, B6, folate, potassium, magnesium, and fibers. However, starchy vegetables are considered a complex carbohydrate. On average, ½ cup of any of the above list contains about 15 grams of carbohydrates, about 80 calories and about 1-3 grams of proteins which breaks down to be a source of quick energy molecule. Starchy vegetables will be digested by the gastric amylase, a digestive enzyme found in the gastrointestinal tract.

The process of complex carbohydrates digestion is long, and it takes several hours before the carbohydrates turn into a sugar, which is the source of our cellular energy fuel.

One of my clinical pearls is that most individuals who have had a hard time losing weight tend to eat large amounts of starchy vegetables a day. This creates a sugar intake imbalance which adds up to more calories than they need. Many lack the digestive enzyme amylase which breaks down the starchy vegetables by breaking the alpha bond releasing glucose. [*23]

Starchy Vegetables If You Are Pre-Diabetic or Diabetic

Many studies prove that high insulin will lead to depletion of zinc, magnesium, and many more minerals and vitamins and will put you at a greater risk of diabetic complications. Starchy vegetables are high on the glycemic index. The glycemic index is an index that measures how fast the food you eat increases your blood sugar. The index rate is in between zero to 100. Safe food will be below 60 on the glycemic index and serving size will be no more than ½ cup. To control your blood sugar, you also want to keep a five hours gap between any starchy vegetable meal.

To make it easy on you I decided to include only the vegetable section of the Glycemic Index so you can choose safe vegetables to control your blood sugar.

GLYCEMIC INDEX - VEGETABLES

Vegetables	Glycemic Index score	Carbohydrates in grams (100g)	GI type
Artichoke	15	2	low
Asparagus	14	1.5	low
Beet	63	8	high
Bell Peppers	10	2.5	low

Vegetables	Glycemic Index score	Carbohydrates in grams (100g)	GI type
Broccoli	10	1.5	low
Brussels sprouts	16	4	Low-med
Cabbage	10	2.5	low
Carrot	70	7	high
Cauliflower	15	2.5	low
Celery	15	1	low
Eggplant	15	3	low-med
Green Beans	14	3.5	low-med
Lettuce(average)	10	1.7	low
Mushroom	10	0.5	low
Onion	10	4	Low-med
Parsnip	98	11	high
Potato, boiled	56	16.5	high
Potato Sweet	50	20	high
Snow Peas	15	4.7	low-med
Spinach	15	3.64	low-med
Tomato	15	3.98	low-med
Zucchini	15	3.5	low-med
Yam	50	32	low-med

Starchy Vegetables and Your GUT Connection

A high starchy vegetables intake in combination with digestive systems challenges, in most individuals will create one or multiple reactions like: **bloating, burping, nausea, heartburn, smelly gas, yeast overgrowth, candida, fatigue, diarrhea and/ or constipation, skin problems, food and environmental allergies, poor memory, joint pain, food craving, and weight gain.** Carbohydrates that are not breaking down properly are fermented in our colon, causing inflammation, irritation, and toxicity. [*2,9,12] Evaluation of digestive enzymes by a professional nutritionist is required to support the needs of your body so that food will be digested properly, regardless of whether it is gluten-free, non-GMO, or organic.

Sue, a software engineer in one of the top successful companies in the Bay Area, contacted me two years ago. She is a tiny woman at 5' foot tall, 170 Pounds. In her early fifties, she has an empty nest and is stressed. She was on a gluten-free diet for 24 months, exercises on a regular basis, and still gained weight regardless of her dietary changes. She was wired, tired, frustrated, irritated, and totally confused with how her body responded – which was entirely different from what she expected. After my nutritional evaluation, I suspected imbalances with the digestive enzymes production, along with food allergies. On a deeper investigation, doing delayed food allergy testing and stool analysis the results showed that she was sensitive to dairy (casein and whey) and egg whites, though the wheat gluten did not come up positive. She had candida albicans infection. Sue needed to change her diet. She needed to cut back on dairy and egg whites, but not gluten. She was put on an antifungal protocol for 90 days with full support to improve her gastrointestinal tract by adding digestive enzymes, probiotics, and other herbs. It was amazing to see how fast she could lose her additional weight and reach her ideal weight, which she still maintains now. Sue has become a great referral source for me.

Enjoy the nutritional benefits of starchy vegetables. Do not avoid eating them, but limit your quantities of starchy vegetables to ½ **cup as a serving size in one meal**. If you do experience any digestion challenges, take it seriously and support your gut with digestive enzymes so you can get the nutrients your body needs to keep your balance. Most digestive enzyme supplements break down in the stomach, and the stomach acid will "kill" 80% of the enzymes. You want to choose enzymes that break down in the colon, so you get the maximum benefits of the product to create the balance. These supplements are much more expensive, though they are effective. Don't save on your health. Support your health, balance, and thrive.

Eat up to ½ cup of starchy vegetables as a serving size in one meal If you are pre-diabetic or diabetic, you should consume less starchy vegetables per meal

GRAINS, BEANS AND LEGUMES

Grains, beans and legumes are high-value foods that you want to eat even if you are on a weight loss program. In general, grains, beans, and legumes will provide us with carbohydrates, proteins, fibers, and minerals like calcium, iron, magnesium, and potassium, along with the vitamins B1, B3, B5, B6 folate, and the trace minerals zinc, copper, phosphorus, and manganese.

Like grains that contain prolamines, lectins, and phytic acid, beans give our bodies some difficulties in digestion. As was discussed earlier, studies show that soaking, sprouting, and fermenting grains prior to cooking will reduce these toxins by 50%. More so, soaking and sprouting eases the ability of the digestion system to digest them. [33,37] Taking simple actions like soaking your beans prior to cooking will save lots of trouble and maintain your nutrient levels.

The ideal serving size of cooked grains, beans, or legumes will be up to ½ cup.

Yes, quantities of these foods are important for losing weight since they are high in calories. One cup of cooked lentils equals about 230 calories. Soy will provide you with about 290 calories. Cooked garbanzo beans will be about 260 calories per one cup. No doubt, these foods will nourish you, and you will want to consume them in moderation, especially if you are looking to lose weight. At the same time, you want to listen to your body and recognize any digestive challenges when eating these foods: **gas, bloating, heartburn, and fatigue** will be some of the symptoms your body will express when having digestion challenges and high blood sugar. Supporting your gut is very important in addition to limiting the quantities consumed of grains, beans, and legumes. Most of my clients face digestion challenges that affect their metabolism and contribute to their weight gain. Once balanced, the weight will come down.

Cooked grains, beans, or legumes: up to ½ cup per serving

THE CHALLENGES WE HAVE EATING FRUITS

Fruits are a great source of vitamins, minerals, antioxidants, fibers, and sugars. Fruits carry two types of sugars: glucose and fructose. We need glucose to fuel our cells. This is the primary source of our energy production cycle. Fructose is a different story.

Most individuals eat more sugar and fructose together than they need. Year-round availability of fruit in addition to juicing, flavored water, soda, sport drinks, sweetened drinks, and dried fruits contribute to a health hazard. Sugar is added even to baby formulas. The average American consumes ½ pound of sugar a day which equals to be about 180 pounds of sugar a year. These numbers are unbelievably high if you stop for a second and think about it.

Natural fructose from fruits and honey was for decades a great source of energy. The challenges are the quantities of sugar we consume and the fact that our bodies metabolize fructose differently from glucose, which leads to further challenges. Fructose metabolizes only in the liver and it's **not** a source of energy for our cells. Therefore, an excess of fructose puts extra burdens on our liver. To get rid of fructose, the liver needs to convert it to fat. That leads to a condition called insulin resistance where the body produces insulin, but does not use it effectively. As a result, glucose builds up rather than being used as a source of energy. The excess of sugar will lead to metabolic syndrome diseases such as diabetic hypertension, lipidemia, and obesity.

Fructose may create liver toxicity the same as over consuming alcohol that turns to ethanol. They both produce oxidative damage to our cells, which leads to inflammation and chronic diseases that are associated with inflammation. Increased uric acid levels can lead to gout and kidney stones and high blood pressure. This can lead to gut dysbiosis, yeast and bacteria over growth, hormonal imbalances, brain dysfunction, and obesity.

Hundreds of studies have shown the vicious cycle of over consumption of sugar. Facts speak for themselves – over consumption of sugar will challenge our health, even if the source is gluten-free.

Natural fructose in small amounts, up to 50 grams per day, which is about ½ cup is the ideal consumption of fructose. For those who are already challenged by high blood sugars or having gut issues, the serving size needs to be reduced to ¼ of a cup. Yes, that much. My best advice here is to limit your sugar intake even if the source is healthy like a fresh, organic apple.

Eat ¼ to ½ cup of fruit a day as a serving size

FRUCTOSE IS NOT HIGH FRUCTOSE CORN SYRUP

Fructose from fruits are not the same as high fructose corn syrup. The ratio between sugars and fructose in high fructose corn syrup is 45% to 55%. Most commercially processed food (including gluten-free) will add high fructose corn syrup to "enrich" the flavor and make us crave it.

We consume about 180 pounds of sugar a year with 63 pounds of it being high fructose corn syrup. Among young adolescents the numbers are even worse – 12% of their total caloric intake daily comes from fructose alone, which is 73 grams of fructose per day. Seven out of ten children will be obese by the time they turn 18 years old. The health consciousness of our present and future generation is a disaster. Nutrition, specifically better food choices in small amounts, is the only way to change it. [*28]

EVEN HEALTHY SOURCES OF FRUITS, STARCHY VEGETABLES BEANS AND GRAINS ARE SUGARS

Fruits, starchy vegetables, beans and grains are all great and healthy sources of foods. At the end of the digestion process each group of the foods as mentioned earlier breaks down into simple sugars (a different type of sugar, though still sugar). The process is completed by digestive enzymes that break the bonds between the sugar molecules turning it into simple sugars.

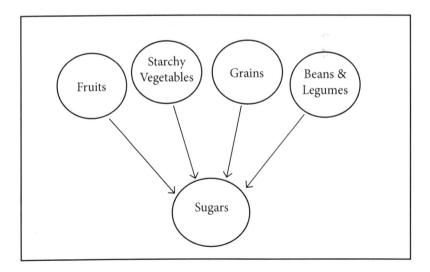

Over-consuming healthy sources of these four groups of foods will affect your blood sugar levels, challenge your digestive system, and create inflammation and weight gain. **The truth is that you want to consume healthy sources of carbohydrates and sugars in moderation.** The goal is to keep your blood sugar levels balanced. Our blood sugar fluctuates daily. Many factors contribute to your blood sugar fluctuations on top of what you eat. Factors like sleep, hormones, medications, stress, and physical activity can affect your blood sugar. It's never static. A healthy range will be in between 80-90mg/dL. These physiological processes are dependent on the food - "fuel" we eat. The balance between nutrients ingested during the "active period" provides fuel for energy to the cells. The fuel stored during the "resting and fasting periods" maintain sustainable metabolic homeostasis. [18] This delicate point will create normal blood sugar fluctuations and can be seen as a paradigm of the circadian control of energy metabolism. [31] If your job demands physical challenges like bending, climbing, walking, crawling, or standing then you need to add extra calories to meet the energy expenditure. If you exercise at least one hour three times a week, you need to increase food intake to meet your body's needs. So now it is your choice to make. What kind of food will you supply to support your body's need for energy? If this question is ignored, you will lose control, you will crave more carbs and sweets, blood sugar will go up, inflammation will be created, and you will gain weight. **Listen to the needs of your body, and supply healthy food that will carry you to balanced health and weight.**

HOW MUCH LESS WILL BE CONSIDER HEALTHY AND BALANCED?

The formula to achieve better and healthy carbohydrate and sugar levels was designed after hours of clinical experience working with many of my clients who wished to lose weight, like you. The formula is: healthy serving size, frequency, and combination of one or more of the foods.

So, let's dive into **The "Balance Diet Formula":**

	Fruit	Starchy Vegetables	Beans (*1)	Grains (gluten and gluten-free grains)
Serving Size (*2)	¼- ½ cup	¼- ½ cup	¼- ½ cup	¼- ½ cup
Frequency	Every 4 hours	Every 4 hours	Every 4 hours	Every 4 hours
Eat each Group of Food Separately	√	√	√	√
Snacks	Vegetables, Fats and/or proteins	Vegetables, Fats and/or proteins	Vegetables, Fats and/or proteins	Vegetables, Fats and/or proteins

* 1 - Beans are also considered to be plant based proteins (look at this section as well)

* 2 - Serving size - **(depends on your health starting point, and if you are vegetarian)**

* if you are found to have **food sensitives or allergies AVOID** these foods even if it's a healthy food

Serving size –To balance your carbohydrate and sugar intake, you want to keep the serving size of up to ¼ to ½ cup of any of the sub groups mentioned above. If you have diabetes or if you fight a chronic inflammatory disease like heart disease, cancer, autoimmune disease: MS, Colitis, Crohn's or Rheumatoid Arthritis (RA), you want to stay on the lower range of the formula and SHOULD NOT go above ½ cup as your balanced, healthy serving size. There is no one-size-fits-all nutrition plan. This is general information, and it's NOT designed for you specifically. You should always consult with a professional nutritionist to formulate a plan for meeting your carbohydrate and sugar needs which must be done based on your starting point health.

Frequency – This depends on food sources. But first, let's distinguish between: **real food** (whole dense, fresh, organic) and **commercially-processed food.**

- <u>**If real food**</u> – You want to wait four hours between each meal that includes any of the sub foods.

- <u>**If commercially-processed food**</u> - You want to consume no more than **five grams of net carbohydrates every four hours (even if its gluten-free food).**

The reason you want to create this time-frame gap is to control your blood sugar and insulin levels, improve your metabolism, reduce inflammation, and lose weight. To do so, you want to know how to calculate your net carbohydrates from commercially-processed food.

WHAT ARE NET CARBOHYDRATES AND HOW DO I CALCULATE THEM?

Net carbohydrates are the grams of your total carbohydrate food sources minus the fibers and the sugars. Some products will add "sugar alcohol" and/or "glycerin," which needs to be subtracted as well, so you can get the accurate net carbohydrate amount.

For example: ½ cup of gluten-free crackers include 24 grams of total carbohydrates, 3 grams of fibers, and 2 grams of sugars. Your net carbohydrates is 18 grams (24-3-3=18 grams).

Total Carbohydrates:	24 grams
Fibers:	(3) grams (minus)
Sugars:	(2) grams (minus)
Net Carbohydrates:	18 grams

In this example, regardless of how healthy the food source is - 18 grams of net carbohydrates are three times more than what your body needs to balance your sugar levels, especially, if you are diabetic or dealing with chronic inflammatory disease.

Preparing your foods will help you to minimize the "loss of control" effect, and it will improve your quality of life. So many of my clients are working in high-tech companies in the Bay Area, California. The food is free and considered to be healthy and still so many suffer from being overweight and having high cholesterol and high blood sugar. Any efforts you take to increase your home-made food will support your health. However, I totally understand that in this hectic and stressful lifestyle we are all living, there is no other way but dining out once in a while. If you buy ready to go foods, you want to check **food labels,** you want to keep the **five grams of net carbohydrates every four hours,** and **plan your meals.** If you eat more than five grams (which you are likely to do), try to eat it in the **first part of the day** (no later than 4pm), so you can burn some of the energy and not convert it into fat.

HERE IS A CONVENIENT NET CARBOHYDRATES INDEX:

Apple = 17.4 net carbs	Cantaloupe balls 1/2 cup = 6.7 net carbs	ASPARAGUS Steamed 4 spears = 1.6 net carbs	Collard Greens steamed 1 cup = 4.0 net carbs
Apricots- 6 fresh whole = 18.4 net carbs	Honeydew balls 1/2 cup = 7.3 net carbs	Green Beans steamed 1/2 cup = 2.9 net carbs	Corn Kernels 1/2 cup = 12.6 net carbs
California Hass Avocado = 3.4 net carbs	Watermelon balls 1/2 cup = 5.1 net carbs	Yellow Wax, steamed 1/2 cup = 2.9 net carbs	Cucumber slices 1/2 cup = 1.0 net carbs
Florida Avocado = 11.0 net carbs	Orange Whole = 12.9 net carbs	Bok Choy 1/2 cup = 0.2 net carbs	Broiled Eggplant 1 cup = 4.2 net carbs
Banana (small) = 21.2 net carbs (skip the Bananas)	Papaya 1/2 = 6.1 net carbs		Endive 1/2 cup = 0.4 net carbs

Blackberries 1 cup = 10.8 net carbs	Peach whole = 7.2 net carbs	Broccoli 1/2 cup = 2 net carbs	Fava Beans 1/2 cup = 12.1 net carbs
Blueberries 1 cup = 14.6 net carbs	Pineapple fresh chunks 1/2 cup = 8.7 net carbs	Broccoli Rabe 1/2 cup = 2.0 net carbs	Fennel fresh 1/2 cup = 1.8 net carbs
Cherries 1 cup = 17 net carbs	Pomegranate 1/4 cup = 6.4 net carbs	Broccolini 1/2 cup = 6.7 net carbs	Garlic fresh 1 clove = 0.9 net carbs
Cranberries whole 1 cup = 8.0 net carbs	Raisins (golden) 1 tbs = 7.8 net carbs	Brussel Sprouts steamed 1/2 cup = 4.7 net carbs	Jicama raw 1/2 cup = 2.5 net carbs)
Dates - 1/2 chopped = 59.0 net carbs (skip the dates)	Raisins (seedless) 1 tbs = 7.4 net carbs	Green Shredded uncooked 1/2 cup = 1.1 net carbs	Kale steamed 1 cup = 4.2 net carbs
Grapefruit whole = 15.6 net carbs	Raspberries 1 cup = 6.0 net	Green Cabbage steamed 1/2 cup = 1.6 net carbs	Lettuce Boston Bibb 1 cup = 0.8 net carbs
Grapes (green/seedless) 1 cup = 27.0 net carbs (High in net carbs!)	Strawberries 1 cup = 6.8 net carbs	Red Cabbage uncooked 1/2 cup = 1.4 net carbs	Iceberg 1 cup = 0.4 net carbs
	Tangerine small = 6.2 net carbs	Savoy Cabbage steamed 1/2 cup = 1.9 net carbs	Romaine 1 cup = 0.4 net carbs
	ARTICHOKES Whole = 6.9 net carbs	Whole raw 1 large carrot = 6.5 net carbs	Mushroom - Portabello 4oz. = 4.1 net carbs
Grapes (purple) 1 cup = 14.8 net carbs	Hearts marinated 4 pieces = 2.0 net carbs	Sliced, steamed = 5.6 net carbs	Shitake Cooked 1/2 cup = 8.8 net carb
Guava 1/2 cup = 5.3 net carbs		Yucca cooked 1/2 cup = 26.0 net carbs	Straw in a jar or can 1/2 cup = 2.0 net carbs
Kiwi whole = 8.7 net carbs		Raw Cauliflower 1/2 cup = 1.4 net carbs	Button or white mushrooms 1/2 cup = 1.4 net carbs
Mango 1/2 cup = 12.5 net carbs		Steamed Cauliflower 1 cup = 1.8 net carbs	Mustard Greens steamed 1 cup = 0.2 net carbs

Yes, you have four grams (0.14oz) of net carbohydras in one cup of steamed broccoli. However, the nutritional benefits to your body out of one cup of broccoli are extremely high – much higher than ½ cup of gluten-free crackers at the same net carbohydrates levels.

What You Want To Do:

✓ Read Labels.

✓ Consume no more than five grams of net. carbohydrates every four hours.

✓ Eat net carbohydrates in the first part of the day

✓ Plan your meals.

✓ **Cook your OWN FOOD if possible for as many meals as you can.**

EAT EACH SUB GROUP SEPARATELY

If you eat each sub group (fruits, starchy vegetables, beans, and grains) separately in the suggested serving size, you will be able to keep your blood sugar levels and calorie intake balanced. It will also improve your metabolism and digestion, reduce self-fermentation processes (which will be presented as gases and bloating), reduce self-production of sugar alcohol, and reduce inflammation. Therefore, you will lose weight.

Symptoms like smelly gas, bloating, indigestion, craving for sweets and carbs, moodiness, brain fogginess, fatigue, and weight gain are a presentation of over consuming foods that turn into sugar even if they are considered a healthy food source. These body reactions may feed your gut bacteria and elevate your body's acidity and toxicity, thus slowing you down on your goal to lose weight. MODERATION is the KEY for Balanced Weight.

ADOPT THESE SET OF RULES AND SEE AMAZING RESULTS ON YOUR SCALE.

Additional Information:

1. Grains that have been milled and refined, gluten of gluten-free – where the bran and the germ have been removed have a higher glycemic index compared to whole grains.

2. Finely ground grains will be digested quicker due to the higher level of fibers.

3. Fruits and vegetables tend to have higher levels of sugars.

4. Meals that have healthy fats and acid like lemon or apple cider vinegar will be converted into sugar slower.

THE VALUE OF EATING SNACKS

Snacks are as important as any other of your three "big" meals, breakfast, lunch or dinner. We need snacks for balancing and maintaining our energy production as well as blood sugar levels throughout the day.

Most individuals will skip snacks, thinking that by avoiding eating snacks they will be able to cut down on their calorie intake and as a result, they will lose weight quicker. The truth is just the opposite. Studies demonstrate that individuals who cut down on snacks prior to a meal will eat a larger size meal to close the gap of calories needed and the chances that they will "lose control" on the quantity of the food is higher. [*11,24] So basically, if you skip snacks you will eat larger amounts of food, but the quality of your food choices will decline. Most likely, you will choose finger foods, fast foods, pizza, and sandwiches which will affect your weight.

Include snacks as part of your daily food intake. Don't miss this opportunity to **NOURISH** your body on the cellular level. Eat **vegetables** and/or healthy **fats** and/or **proteins** for snacks or a **combination** of 2 or 3 of the food choices.

Preparation and planning are your keys for a successful and healthy weight loss program which must include healthy snacks.

Some Snacks Ideas:

- Box small portions of your **leftover meals** as your healthy snacks
- Fill a zip lock bag with **fresh organic veggies** for the next 3-4 working days
- Bag small portions (up to 20 units overall) of raw **nuts and seeds**
- (Please note: over eating nuts and seeds may increase your calories intake and cause weight gain especially if you don't exercise regularly)
- ½ fresh **avocado**
- Packaged **salads** (if you do not have the time to create your own)
- **Hummus** with celery sticks (or any other vegetables)
- Half a pepper stuffed with **tuna or chicken salad**
- 1 hardboiled **egg** with ¼ cup of cherry tomatoes (or any other vegetable)
- **1 apple** (or any other fruit in a small amount)

Snacks are an opportunity for us to leverage our vitamin and mineral intake by eating real foods. It is also an opportunity to balance our blood sugar levels. **Eating small, frequent, high quality snacks, 3 times a day** will reduce levels of hunger and increase satisfaction so you can eat less calories in your next big meal and reduce your weight on the scale.

EATING HEALTHY FATS

Most individual will cut back on fats when they are starting a weight loss program. Avocado, nuts, and seeds, wild caught fish, organic-grass feed meat, olives, eggs, liquid oils, and solid fats like butter, lard, and ghee are all part of your healthy fat food sources which you want to consume in moderation.

Fats are a crucial source for your health. They are essential for energy production and transporting fat soluble vitamins like vitamin A, D, E, and K. Fats support the conversion of carotenes into vitamin A and help balance your hormonal signals. Also, fats support the immune system, improve bone density, support calcium levels, brain, and cognitive functionality, improve metabolism, and offer protection to the heart.

Skipping eating healthy fats in your diet is a big mistake most individuals will make while trying to lose weight. It is true that fats are high in calories (9 calories per gram compared to 4 calories per gram in proteins and carbohydrates), though you need it to balance your energy production, especially if you are cutting back on gluten foods.

You want to focus on healthy fats like monounsaturated and polyunsaturated fats. Avoid consuming the hydrogenated trans fats that the food industry uses on a massive level. Hydrogenation is a process that turns liquid fats into solid form to prevent rancidity and therefore, it prolongs the shelf-life of the product. The challenge with the hydrogenation process is that will create inflammation, increase cholesterol LDL levels, slow down your ability to lose weight, and risk your health. [*26]

Weight loss occurs in cycles. Each cycle may increase oxidation and inflammation levels. To reduce oxidation and inflammation levels, you need to consume more healthy fat foods along and supplement with Omega-3, which will provide proper nutrients to support the immune system. This will reduce body fat, especially fat oxidation in areas such as the adipose tissue, the liver, cardiac, intestinal, and skeletal muscle tissue. This allows the process of weight loss to continue. [*4,5,6,7,10,15,25,29,32,39.]

Even from a cellular energy production perspective, we need to consume fats along with carbohydrates and proteins. The Kreb's Cycle, which is the cellular powerhouse of the mitochondria, is dependent on these three crucial macronutrients. In between 20% and 35% of our daily energy production is based on dietary fats. This cycle is the **only way** fats are used in the energy production pathway. The quality and the quantities of fats are valued to our health and our weight. The ideal ratio of Omega-3 to Omega-6 fats is 2:1. That means that we need to eat about as twice as much Omega-3 as Omega-6. Additionally, it is important to incorporate balanced proportions and healthy sources of fats of essential and non-essential fatty acids, thus maintaining our overall health and sustaining stable weight.

FOOD SOURCES OF OMEGA 3-6-9:

Omega 3 Essential Fatty acids (ALA - Alpha-linolenic acid)	Omega 6 Essential Fatty Acids (AA - Arachidonic acid)	Omega 9 Foods rich in Oleic Acid
• Cold water high fat fish like: wild salmon, sardines, anchovies, mackerel, shad, herring and trout • Flaxseed oil, flaxseeds, flaxseed meal • Hempseed oil, hempseeds • Walnut oil, walnuts • Pumpkin seeds • Brazil nuts • Sesame seeds • Avocado • Coconut oil • Some dark green leafy vegetables like: kale, spinach, mustard greens, collards	• Flaxseed oil, flaxseeds, flaxseed meal • Hempseed oil, hempseeds • Grapeseed oil • Pumpkin seeds • Pignolia (pine) nuts • Pistachio nuts • Sunflower seeds (raw) • Borage oil • Evening primrose oil • Black currant seed oil • Acai • Peanut Oil • Meat • Eggs • Dairy Products	• Olive oil (extra virgin or virgin), olives • Avocados • Almonds • Peanuts • Sesame oil • Pecans • Pistachio nuts • Cashews • Hazelnuts • Macadamia
	Corn, safflower, sunflower, soybean, and cottonseed oils are also sources of Omega 6, but are considered as refined and may be deficient in nutrients	

High quality and healthy fats in small amounts will balance the needs of your body better in the long run and help maintain your goal to lose weight. It's all about being balanced and fats are part of the equation.

> **High quality and healthy fats in small amounts will Balance your body**

HOW MUCH PROTEIN SHOULD YOU EAT?

Unless you are vegan or vegetarian, eating meat protein is crucial for your health. Protein is a macro nutrient composed of amino acids that is necessary for a proper growth, maintenance, and reparation of the human body's tissues. Proteins are also part of a healthy and balanced immune system, hormones, brain functionality, and enzyme production.

Most studies reveal that a high quality of protein, low in healthy fats and high in vegetables intake diet, will be your best and safest way to lose weight. Moreover, studies show that individuals who ate more protein over a course of 12 weeks felt more satisfied and lost 11 pounds overall, which was 2 pounds more than those who ate only one portion of protein a day. Also, it boosted their metabolism by up to 80 to 100 calories per day, compared to lower protein diets. [17,30,35,36,38,40]

The Recommended Dietary Allowance (RDA) for protein is a modest 0.8 of protein per 1 kilogram of body weight (1 kg = 2.2 lbs.) or 0.36 grams per pound. This amount takes you to 56 grams per day for the average sedentary man and 46 grams per day for the average sedentary woman. Obviously, if you are an athlete, you need more protein compared to an individual who exercises twice a week for 1 hour each time. An athlete will need about 0.5 – 0.65 grams per pound, or 1.4 – 1.8 grams per kg. If you are post-surgery or if you are pregnant or breastfeeding, the need for protein will change [8,22,27]

Your weight and your health's starting point are significant contributors for the grams of protein per day you need to eat.

How do I calculate grams of proteins for a healthy average adult needs?

If your body weight is 140 pounds you want to divide this number by 2.2 and then multiply it by .8 to get the grams of protein you need per day.

For example: 140/2.2 = 63.6 x .8 = 50 grams of protein per day

Recommended Daily Protein Intake

The average adult needs	Strength training athlete's needs	Endurance athletes needs	Adult In Healing Process
Approx. 0.8 grams per kilogram (2.2lbs) of body weight per day	Approx. 1.4 to 1.8 grams per kilogram (2.2lbs) of body weight per day	Approx. 1.2 to 1.4 grams per kilogram (2.2lbs) of body weight per day	Approx. 0.45 to 0.6 grams per pound of body weight per day

GRAMS OF PROTEINS VS. AMOUNT OF PROTEIN IN EACH FOOD

Grams of proteins are not equal to grams of the actual amount of protein in that food. It may be confusing, but let me explain via an example: 4 oz (=100 grams) of salmon fish equals only 26 grams of protein, which said, you can have about 8 oz of salmon a day to meet the protein requirements if your body weight is 140 pounds. **Are you eating that much?** In my clinical observation, most individuals will have less protein intake than they need. When you cut back on grains, sugars, and carbohydrates, you will get hungrier faster. Most likely, you will lose control, and in less than 21 days you will start gaining back every pound you lost.

It's NOT what you AVOID eating, It's what you DO EAT

LIST OF HIGH-PROTEIN FOODS AND AMOUNT OF PROTEIN IN EACH

Beef	Chicken	Fish	Pork	Eggs and Dairy
Hamburger patty, 4 oz – 28 grams protein	Chicken breast, 3.5 oz - 30 grams protein	Most fish fillets or steaks are about 22-30 grams of protein for 3 ½ oz (100 grams) of cooked fish	Pork chop, average - 22 grams protein	Egg, large - 6 grams' protein
Steak, 6 oz – 42 grams	Chicken thigh – 10 grams (for average size	Tuna, 6 oz can - 40 grams of protein	Pork loin or tenderloin, 4 oz – 29 grams	Milk, 1 cup - 8 grams
Most cuts of beef 7 grams of protein per ounce	Drumstick – 11 grams		Ham, 3 oz serving – 19 grams	Cottage cheese, ½ cup - 15 grams

Beef	Chicken	Fish	Pork	Eggs and Dairy
	Wing – 6 grams Chicken meat, cooked, 4 oz – 35 grams		Ground pork, 1 oz raw – 5 grams; 3 oz cooked – 22 grams	Yogurt, 1 cup – usually 8-12 grams, check label Soft cheeses (Mozzarella, Brie, Camembert) – 6 grams per oz
			Bacon, 1 slice – 3 grams	Medium cheeses (Cheddar, Swiss) – 7 or 8 grams per oz
				Hard cheeses (Parmesan) – 10 grams per oz

THE QUANTITY AND QUALITY OF YOUR PROTEIN SOURCE DOES MATTER

Protein requirements have been revised by the medical community more than one time throughout the history of the science of nutrition from 100 to 120 grams per day to 20 to 30 grams a day. I honestly believe that today with so many protein choices we have such as meat, fish, dairy, and eggs, the protein allowance is around 70 to 90 grams per day on average. Remember the quantities of your protein intake vary and depend on your gender, levels of activity, health starting point, stress, and more. On top of protein quantities, the quality of the protein sources you consume counts as well. In general, my best suggestion is that one should choose grass fed, organic, and non-GMO products as much as possible, especially when we are talking about commercially processed food. Our food is far from the original form in which it was designed. To prolong the shelf-life and improve taste, the food industry includes additives.

The following is a partial list of additives added into our food **which we should try to avoid:**

- Aldrin
- Benzene
- Butylated Hydroxyanisole - BHA (E-319)
- Butylated Hydroxytoluene – BHT – (E-320)
- Tertiry-Butyl Hydroquinone – BHTQ (E321)
- Bisphenol A – BHT (E-321)
- Chlordane
- DDT
- Dieldrin
- Heptachlor
- Hexachloride
- Lindane
- Methoxychlor
- Monosodium glutamate – MSG (E621)
- Nitrates
- Nitrites
- Stilbestrol
- Sex hormones: bovine growth hormone (rBST/rBGH)
- Toxaphene
- Blue #1 – Bright Blue, Brilliant Blue
- Blue #2 – Royal Blue, Indigotine
- Green #3 – Sea Green, Fast Green
- Red #3 - Cherry Red, Erythrosine
- Red #40 – Orange Red, Allura Red
- Yellow #5 – Lemon Yellow, Tatrazine
- Yellow #6 – Orange, Sunset Yellow

In addition, hormones, antibiotics, and prolonged lactation challenges the gastric process, our hormonal signals, creates inflammation, and causes weight gain.

Read Labels! Don't get fooled by misleading advertisements, be a SMART shopper!

Chose **Clean, Grass Fed, Organic** and **non-GMO** products
Free of Hormones and Free of Antibiotic

as much as you can afford

HIGH PROTEIN DIET

Keep in mind that a high protein diet without enough green vegetables and fruits to balance alkaline-acidity-and-toxins ratio, will destroy the glandular system. Thus, it will overstress the liver, adrenals, and kidneys. Even protein supplements can throw off the balance we need. Protein powders are made from fragmented foods like soy, rice, dried eggs, Brewer's yeast, barley, whey milk, and malt. Fragmented foods tend to over-load the body with substances which contribute to the uric acid formation (a bio-waste product). Thus, fragmented food adds burden on the body to secrete them.

Meet Jim, he was recently diagnosed with gout. His uric acid levels were 6.5, and his kidneys markers were elevated too. He also suffered from offensive smelly gas, joint pain, and headaches. On the initial consultation, he reported he's using a bodybuilder whey protein 3 times a day. In dramatic fashion, his blood panel results changed after he stopped taking this protein supplements. His inflammation was reduced, his liver detoxification and digestion improved, and he corrected his nutritional deficiencies by eating more vegetables, fruits, nuts, and seeds. After six months in the program, he went from high risk gout to normal. Balanced protein intake was for him and so many others a key for Balanced Health.

To make your life easy, you want to have in between 3 and 5 portions of protein a day. This is a good rule of thumb you want to follow, so your body will get enough amino acids, which are your body's building blocks. Make sure you diversify the sources of proteins you eat as well.

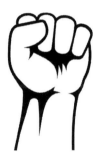

Eating proteins (that is non-GMO, clean, grass fed, free of antibiotic, free of pesticides, and free hormones) is crucial for your health. Yes, the quality of your meat, fish, eggs, and dairy should be part of any healthy and balanced diet. You have to remember that **eating high amounts of dairy products and commercial meat high in antibiotics, pesticides, and hormones means those things will accumulate in your body.** Studies linked "non-clean" proteins to obesity and chronic diseases such as heart, kidney, arthritis, and cancer. Make sure you eat clean, organic, grass fed proteins as much as you can afford in order to support your health and to keep you Balanced. **Always include vegetables with any meat protein to balance your pH levels.**

PLANT BASE PROTEIN SOURCES

Plant based proteins are a great option to diversify your protein intake. You should enjoy eating more than one source of proteins. Yes, eggs, dairy, fish and meat are complete proteins in the sense that they provide you with all 20 different amino acids. Also, they contain the nine essential amino acids that are needed from food because the human body can't produce it. However, plant-base proteins do contain a wide variety of amino acids including the nine essential amino acids, but they are also high in their calories volume.

We have three major groups of plant based protein aside from vegetables: beans, grains (gluten and gluten free), and nuts and seeds.

Plant Based Protein Beans

One gram of plant based protein is equal to 10.4 calories. For example: 1 cup of cooked kidney beans (= 172 grams by weight) will provide you with about 14 grams of proteins, which is about 145.6 calories (14 x 10.4 =145.6 calories).

Yes, plant based protein are great source of food, which you want to include in your diet. Just remember that if you want to lose weight and/or you struggle with high blood sugar and high cholesterol levels, you want to limit the serving size to ½ cup every 4 hours as was mentioned in the Balance formula.

Below is a list of high plant base protein beans sources to calorie ratio that you can enjoy eating:

Protein source in 100g	1 cup cooked (about 172g by weight) Grams changes based on food source and quality if (organic, Non-GMO etc.)	Use	Protein to Calorie Ratio
Kidney Beans Gluten Free	17g	• Alternative to rice, pasta or beef and fish • Can be served alone or over vegetables and greens • Can be served cold/hot • Great for soups	About 176.4
White Beans Gluten Free	17g	• Alternative to rice, pasta or beef and fish • Can be served alone or over vegetables and greens • Can be served cold/hot • Great for soups	About 176.4
Soy Beans Gluten Free Note: If possible, buy/eat organic and non GMO soy	17g	• Alternative to rice, pasta or beef and fish • Can be served alone or over vegetables and greens • Good base for a veggie burger • Great for soups • Can be served cold/hot	About 176.4

Lima Beans Gluten Free	15g	• Can be served alone or over vegetables and greens, rice, quinoa and pasta • Great for soups • Can be served cold or hot	About 156
Fava Beans Gluten Free	14g	• Can be served alone or over vegetables and greens, rice, quinoa and pasta • Great for soups • Can be served cold or hot	About 145.6
Black Beans Gluten Free	15g	• Can be served alone or over vegetables and greens, rice, quinoa and pasta • Great for soups • Can be served cold or hot	About 156
Mung Bean Gluten Free	14g	• Can be served alone or over vegetables and greens, rice, quinoa and pasta • Great for soups • Can be served cold or hot	About 145.6
Lentil Gluten Free	17.9g	• Can be served alone or over vegetables and greens • Great for soups • Can be served cold/ hot	About 186.16
Garbanzo Bean (Hummus) Gluten Free	19.8g	• Great over vegetables and greens, rice, quinoa and pasta • Can be served cold or hot • Great for soups	About 206

Beans are also high in carbohydrates. In general, one serving of ½ cup cooked beans is about 15-25 grams of carbohydrates. This amount of carbohydrates will affect you sugar levels and weight. Also, the way you cook your food and the spices you are adding (if they are fresh or not) are also a significant contributors of hidden carbohydrates, sugars, and calories.

Eat beans in moderation and make sure you are eating more than one type of beans.

You want to remember that most plant-based proteins are high in their caloric intake compared to animal-based proteins. If your intent is to lose weight, you need to monitor your caloric intake differently.

Plant Based Protein Grains

One gram of plant-base protein is equals to about 40 calories. For example: 1 cup of cooked white rice will provide you with about 4.5 grams of proteins which is about 180 calories (4.5 x 40 = 180 calories).

The following table will give you better picture of plant-based protein grains sources:

Protein source	½-1 cup cooked Grams changes based on food source and quality (organic, Non-GMO etc)	Use	Protein to Calorie Ratio
Quinoa, Buckwheat, Rice, Millet, Farro, Amaranth (cooked) Gluten Free	6 -11g Protein / 1 Cup	• Alternative to wheat pasta • Can served alone or over vegetables and greens • Good base for a veggie burger • Can served cold/hot as a cereal breakfast	About 200-250 calories per cup

Seitan Wheat Gluten Note: Seitan is a mix of wheat gluten with herbs and spices. The mix is hydrating with water or stock and than simmering. If you are Celiac or gluten sensitive AVOID it.	24g Protein / 4 Ounces/0.5 cup	• Alternative to beef and fish • Can served alone or over vegetables and greens • Good base for a veggie burger	About 206 calories per cup
Rice Gluten Free	4.5g	• Alternative to beef and fish • Can served alone or over vegetables and greens • Good base for a veggie burger	About 216 calories per cup
Spirulina	6g Protein / 10 grams	• A blue-green algae	1 tablespoon 20 calories

You have to diversify the food sources you are eating. Make sure you are eating more than one type of grain – a gluten or gluten free source.

Plant Based Protein Nuts and Seeds

One gram of plant based protein nuts and seeds is about 15.8 calories. For example: 2 teaspoons of raw almonds, will provide you with about 8 grams of proteins which is about calories (8 x 15.8 = 126.4 calories).

The following table will give you better picture of plant based protein nuts and seeds sources:

Protein source	2-4 Teaspoons • Grams changes based on food source and quality	Use	Protein to Calorie Ratio
Seeds:	5-10g Protein (2-4 teaspoons, Raw) • Chia Seeds (5g) • Flaxseed (8g) • Hemp Seeds (10g) • Pumpkin Seeds (8g) • Sunflower Seeds (7g) • Sesame seed (7g)	• Great over vegetables and greens, rice, quinoa and pasta • Better eaten raw	High in calories (*See formula)
Nuts:	3-8g Protein (2-4 teaspoons, Raw) • Almond (8g) • Brazil Nut (5g) • Cashews (5g) • Coconut (3g) • Macadamia (3g) • Pecan (3g) • Peanuts (8g) • Pistachios (6g) • Sunflower Seeds (6g) • Walnut (5g)	• Great over vegetables and greens • Better eaten raw	High in calories (*See formula)

Once again, you have to diversify the food sources you are eating. Make sure you are eating more than one type of nuts and seeds.

You want to remember, that most plant based proteins (nuts and seeds) are high in their caloric intake compared to animal-based proteins.

FINAL THOUGHTS

NUTRITION IS THE "GLUE" BETWEEN OUR MIND, BODY AND SOUL

O UR BODY IS SUCH a complex system that it makes NO sense to me that people are using electronic devices to track their calories, sleep, food intake, and emotions just to name a few. Given the fact that those devices are so popular, I'm asking myself – have we lost the sense of listening to our bodies signals and are we going too far being so scientific? Food is information that carries hundreds of our biological pathways daily. If you are using nutrition as a therapeutic tool to Balance your biochemistry or any labeled disease or underline causes, you must upload yourself for so much more nutrients to create the required Balance. Nutrition is the "glue" between mind, body and spirit. If we eat food that is not "clean" (commercial, processed, and manipulated with so many chemicals, additives, and colors that our bodies can't recognize it any more) as our nutrients, it will lead us to imbalances in more than one body system. Over time, it will lead us to to weight gain and disease. My question is, how are unclean foods helpful? We are harming our bodies, souls, and spirits. Let's build back our core foundations. Optimum wellness is based on nutrition. Making the decision to take this nutritional and therapeutic journey is a very compelling invitation to you:

to create the change and to commit to your spiritual journey. No electronic device can make that change for you. That requires preparations, rituals, and determination to bring back your body-mind-spirit to the center.

Learning the truth about your body's needs is sometimes very scary. Though, reality is so much stronger and more fulfilling. It's either you walk the healthy path, listening to your body and practicing health in every bite you take, or you are falling back. Clarity and honesty are your keys for Balanced health. So many of us are dreaming of the perfect body and the perfect weight. Blocking ourselves from the real cores of our existence is completely dependent on our nutrition. Illness, as common as diabetic or high blood pressure is, a "wake-up" call or, if you will, an opportunity to make the nutritional and the lifestyle changes your body deserves to achieve and maintain Balance. Adopting nutrition is a celebration of Balanced life, regardless the efforts involved in shopping, chopping, and chewing. The energy we are spending when we or someone we love is sick is greater than anything we did before.

Healing can happen on different levels within us, starting with the physical level going through emotional, mental, and spiritual levels. This is the power of proper nutrition. This is the light food can carry. This is the healing power of nutrition, which is the element or if you will the "glue" between mind, body and spirit.

RECIPES

HERE ARE SOME OF my favorite recipes which was proven effective with my clients to achieved Balance and Optimum Health. Please remember that each one of us is unique in his or her way. The starting point, which represent systems imbalances, is different and therefore, it is wise to start with these suggested recipes keeping in mind that you may need further adjustment by a professional for Balance and Optimum Health.

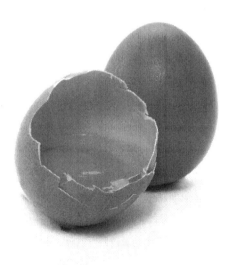

Eggs – Quick and Easy to Make

How Many Eggs a Day Are Good for You?

Eggs are a great source of protein, calcium, vitamins and minerals that are essential for our health.

One large egg contains 78 calories, 6.29g protein, 25mg of calcium, 0.59mg of iron and 112.7mcg of choline. One egg also has folate, vitamin A (260IU), vitamin D (44IU), lutein (176 mcg), zeaxanthin with B-complex vitamins, 6.6 mcg of selenium and 54mg of potassium.

Although eggs contain 22mg of cholesterol, studies show there is no direct correlation between eating eggs and heart disease in adults who have no history of cholesterol problems. In fact, studies show eggs have no effect on blood cholesterol within 70% of the population! The American Heart Association recommends people with high cholesterol to consume no more than one egg a day. A 2006 publication from Harvard Medical School suggests an average of one egg per day for maintaining a healthy cholesterol level. If you have a high cholesterol level, I would recommend eating an egg every other day to stay on the safe side.

As with any food intake, moderation is the key for balanced health. Obviously your daily intake will depend on your health history, age, weight, sex and level of physical activity.

To save some calories, the best way to prepare eggs is boiling them for 5-7 minutes. If you fry your eggs with oil or butter, remember to include the extra calories when calculating your calorie intake! You'll have to do the same if you prepare your eggs using cheese or milk. If you are concerned about your cholesterol, you can eat more of the yolk (the white part). Add vegetables to any scrambled egg breakfast for a healthier way to get ready and enjoy the day!

Here are some delicious, nutritionally rich egg recipes for you to try!

"Shkshukah"

The Perfect Mediterranean Style Sunny-Side Up Egg

(1 serving)

Ingredients:

1 organic onion, chopped

4 organic tomatoes, chopped

1 organic red pepper, chopped

2 organic garlic cloves, chopped

¼ cup fresh organic basil, chopped

¼ cup organic tomato paste

2 organic eggs (per serving)

½ cup feta cheese (goat cheese if possible)

1 teaspoon black pepper

1 teaspoon sunflower oil

Directions:

Preheat oil over medium-high heat in a medium sized pan for 1 minute

Sauté onions, tomatoes, red peppers and garlic until soft

Add tomato paste and stir

Add basil and black pepper, let the mixture boil

Once boiled, reduce heat and cook until the mixture turns thick

Add the eggs into the mixture, cook for 2 minutes

Sprinkle feta cheese on top of the eggs and cover the pan

Cook for 20 minutes on low heat or until excess liquids evaporate

Serve immediately

Dip a fresh slice of bread (or gluten free bread) into your Shakshuka with fresh salad served on the side and enjoy!

Poached Egg with Arugula and Avocado

(1 serving)

Ingredients:

2 fresh organic eggs

½ fresh organic avocado, diced and sliced

¼ cup of sheep or goat feta cheese

½ cup fresh organic onions, chopped

½ cup fresh organic crimini mushrooms, chopped

¼ cup fresh organic arugula, chopped

¼ teaspoon fresh or dry organic oregano
Salt and black pepper to taste

Directions:

Poached Egg:

Fill a saucepan with about 4 inches of water and bring to a boiling point

Reduce the heat and let water simmer (few bubbles)

Crack 1 egg into a small bowl

Gently slip the egg into the simmering water

Cook for about 4 minutes or until egg white is cooked

Gently lift the poached egg out of the saucepan and move to the serving plate.

Vegetables:

Sauté onions and mushrooms with oregano for 2-4 minutes

Add salt and black pepper to taste

Serving Plate:

While the eggs are cooking, set the sliced avocado and cheeses on the serving plate

Add the cooked vegetables and poached egg

Sprinkle arugula on top of the egg

Optional: drizzle 1 teaspoon of olive oil onto the poached egg

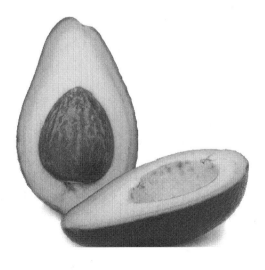

Choose Aluminum FREE Baking Powder

It's available, it's cheap and it's healthier!

Most baking powders are based on the ingredient sodium bicarbonate. When it becomes moistened, it releases carbon dioxide which makes dough rise. Overusing sodium bicarbonate can cause side effects such as frequent urination, headaches, mood swings, muscle pain, slow breathing, fatigue and swelling in the feet.

There are two types of sodium bicarbonate: fast and slow acting. The fast acting powder is activated at room temperature and will be effective a few seconds after getting wet. The slow acting powders will be activated by the oven's heat and will provide a slower rise. In general, about 90% of commercial baking powders have double acting active sodium components containing sodium aluminum sulfate or sodium aluminum phosphate. The side effects of these aluminum based components are huge! Studies have linked neuro-degenerative diseases such as Alzheimer's, ADHD, Parkinson's and Autism to aluminum based acid salt toxicity (1).

Aluminum is also in self-rising flour, food additives, salt, baby formulas, coffee creamers, baked goods, drugs, vaccines, cosmetics, food cans, juice pouches and water bottles. Studies also found that aluminum concentration increases by 10 times in foods such as red meat and chicken when cooked in aluminum foil (2).

Do the best you can to choose aluminum-free products, especially food products! Aluminum-free baking powder is available, cheap and healthier!

References

1. Christopher Exley and Thomas Vickers, Elevated brain aluminium and early onset Alzheimer's disease in an individual occupationally exposed to aluminium, Journal of Medical Case Reports, Volume 8

2. Turhan S., Aluminium contents in baked meats wrapped in aluminium foil, Meat Science. 2006 Dec;74(4):644-7

Scrambled Egg Muffins

(4 servings)

Ingredients:

6 fresh organic eggs, beaten

2 tablespoons almond flour

¼ teaspoon cumin seeds

1 teaspoon baking powder
Salt and black pepper

1 teaspoon grapeseed oil

½ cup of vegetables (* see note), chopped thinly

Optional combinations of vegetables:

onion, mushroom, spinach

onion, parsley, tomatoes

pepper, tomatoes, zucchini

kale, tomatoes, onion

dill, mushroom, pre-cooked cauliflower

Directions:

Beat eggs in a mid-size bowl

Add vegetables, cumin seeds, baking powder and almond flour

Add salt and black pepper to taste

Mix until well combined

Coat muffin cups with grapeseed oil (you can use spray oil too)

Fill ¾ of each muffin cup with the egg-vegetable mix

Bake at 375°F for 10-15 minutes or until a toothpick inserted near the
center of the muffin comes out clean

Note:

(*) Any vegetable combination that fits your taste will work for this recipe.

Green Herbs Scrambled Eggs

(1 serving)

Ingredients:

¼ cup organic green onions, chopped

¼ cup organic parsley, chopped

1 pinch organic thyme

¼ cup goat cheese

1-2 organic eggs, beaten

Salt and black pepper to taste

1-2 teaspoons organic avocado oil

Directions:

Whisk eggs

Add herbs and goat cheese, mix

Heat skillet with oil

Pour in the egg mixture

Mix eggs in skillet until fully cooked

Add salt and black pepper to taste

Serve immediately

Egg Breakfast over Swiss Chard Wrap, Beans, and Pepper

(1 serving)

Ingredients:

2 mid-size organic Swiss chard bunches, pre-washed

2 organic eggs, beaten

½ fresh organic avocado, diced and sliced

¼ cup of Pavilions cheese, shredded

¼ cup organic black beans

¼ cup organic fresh cilantro, chopped

1 small organic fresh tomato, chopped thinly Salt and black pepper to taste

¼ teaspoon organic cumin seeds

1-2 golden Greek pepperoncini, pickled (optional)

2 teaspoons avocado oil

Directions:

Whisk eggs until well mixed

Add cheese, cilantro and cumin; mix

Heat skillet with oil

Pour egg mixture in

Mix eggs in skillet until fully cooked

Lay Swiss chard flat on a serving dish

Fill it with scrambled eggs, avocado, tomatoes, cilantro and beans

Fold the sides of the Swiss chard and roll it

Serve immediately while still warm

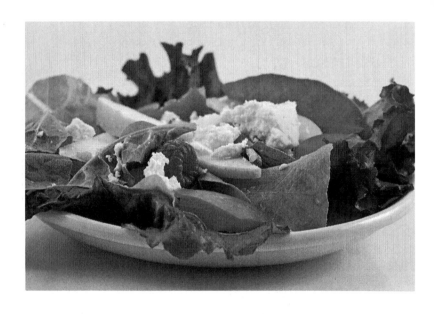

Salads

Most people do not need a nutritionist to tell them eating more salads is a healthy choice to make! However, so many people associate the word "salad" with the idea that it's not going to taste very good. Other people do not understand how filling a salad can actually be when prepared the right way.

Here are some proven salad recipes bursting with flavor while providing your body with the nutrition it needs!

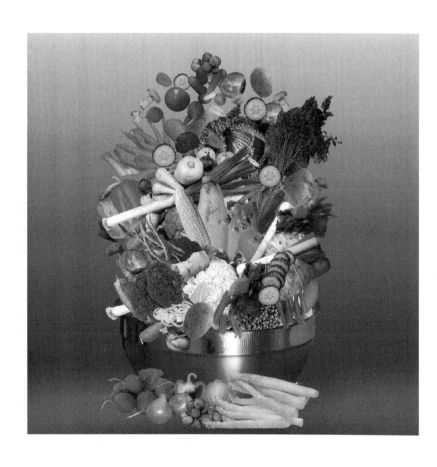

Summer Fresh
Fennel Salads

(1-2 servings)

Ingredients:

2 organic fresh fennel bulbs, sliced thinly crosswise

2 teaspoons of organic cold pressed olive oil

½ cup fresh organic lemon juice
Sea salt to taste

Directions:

Put sliced fennel in a mid-sized bowl

Drizzle with olive oil and lemon juice

Add salt to taste

Let salad stand for 5-10 minutes to allow flavors to meld together

What is Kelp?

Kelp is a super food you definitely should be including in your diet! It is ideal for improving and maintaining an optimal metabolism rate thus supporting healthy weight loss. Kelp is a type of seaweed algae (Phaeophyceae) that is rich in minerals (calcium, potassium, magnesium and iron), trace minerals (copper, selenium and zinc), amino acids (tryptophan, threonine, isoleucine, methionine, cysteine and valine), vitamins (A, B6, B12 and C) as well as iodine which is needed to stimulate a sluggish thyroid.

A healthy and balanced metabolism is supported by our thyroid gland, which helps regulate our weight.

Iodine is the catalyst which starts the metabolic process obtained by nutrition and food supplements. Any challenges on iodine absorption may lead to a compromised thyroid (either hypo or hyperthyroidism). Kelp can be a great source of the iodine needed to boost a sluggish thyroid.

1 cup of kelp noodles only contains 6 calories and 1 gram of carbohydrates! Plus, they can be easily purchased in most health food stores.

Don't wait; make your first kelp salad today!

Here are some delicious, nutritionally rich egg recipes for you to try!

Kelp Noodles, Chinese Cabbage and Kumquats Salads

(1-2 servings)

Ingredients:

2 cups of kelp noodles

1 organic Chinese cabbage, chopped

1 cup organic kumquats (cherry oranges), chopped

1 bundle of organic cilantro, chopped

1 bundle of organic green onion, chopped

2 organic garlic cloves, chopped

2 teaspoons organic sunflower oil

½ cup apple cider vinegar or rice vinegar

½ cup fresh organic lemon juice Kosher salt to taste

Directions:

Rinse noodles in fresh water

Chop kelp noodles into rough chunks and place in a large bowl

Add chopped Chinese cabbage, kumquats, green onion, cilantro and garlic

Season with vinegar, oil, salt and lemon

Mix all ingredients until combined

Kelp Noodles with Tahini Sauce Salad

(1-2 servings)

Ingredients:

2 cups kelp noodles

1 cup raw organic tahini paste (sesame seed paste)

¼ cup Nama shoyu (raw organic soy sauce - (see note)

½ cup fresh organic lemon juice

½ cup water

3 teaspoons apple cider vinegar

½ teaspoon kosher salt

2 organic garlic cloves, chopped

¼ cup nutritional yeast

½ teaspoon powdered turmeric 2 organic zucchinis, chopped

2 bunches of organic kale, steamed

1 cup cherry tomatoes

½ cup organic cilantro, chopped

½ cup organic mint, chopped

½ cup organic green onion, chopped

Directions:

Tahini sauce:

Combine raw tahini, Nama shoyu, lemon, vinegar, water, salt,
nutritional yeast and turmeric

Blend until thick and smooth (add water if necessary)

Rinse noodles in fresh water

Place chopped kelp noodles in a mid-sized bowl

Add zucchini, kale, cherry tomatoes, cilantro and mint; mix

Pour Tahini sauce and mix again

Serve immediately or refrigerate for up to 4 days.

Notes:

(*) If you are sensitive to gluten, you could replace Nama shoyu with a
certified gluten free soy product such as Tamari

(**) If soy sensitive, stir 2 teaspoons of honey with lemon juice, apple
cider vinegar and water instead

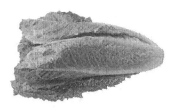

What Do You Know about Napa Cabbage?

Napa cabbage belongs to the powerful family of the cruciferous vegetables, just like cauliflower, broccoli, Brussels sprouts, asparagus, and Bok Choy. You should consume one cruciferous vegetable on a daily basis. If it is not yet included in your daily diet, you should begin with a minimum of 1 cup twice a week and gradually increase your intake to 3-5 cups a week.

Napa cabbage is full of antioxidant and anti-inflammatory substances. It also has glucosinolates that are anti-cancer preventives. Napa cabbage supports the binding process of the digestive system and promotes bile acids to bind with toxins and excrete them out of our body. It may also reduce cholesterol levels.

In 1 cup of raw shredded Napa cabbage there are only 20 calories, 1 gram of protein, 1 gram of fiber, Vitamin C; 46% Recommended Dietary Allowance (RDA), Vitamin A; 26% RDA, Vitamin K; 66.5%; manganese 4.6%, B6; 4.5%; potassium; 3.4% as well as vitamins B1, B2, choline, phosphours, iron, folate, selenium, and niacin.

Napa cabbage can be eaten raw, cooked, and stirred. It is easy to use and I encourage you to include it in your diet. Your body will thank you if you do!

Napa Cabbage, Radishes and Cucumber Salad

(1-2 servings)

Ingredients:

½ organic Napa cabbage, sliced

2-4 organic cucumbers (or 1 English cucumber), sliced

4 green onions, chopped

6 fresh organic radishes, sliced into rings

1 teaspoon sea salt

2 teaspoons sesame oil

2 teaspoons raw black sesame seeds

½ cup apple cider vinegar

Directions:

Mix all ingredients in a large bowl

Let it sit for about 10 minutes

Sprinkle black sesame seeds on top right before serving

Black Lentils, Sweet Potatoes and Pomegranate Seeds Salad

(1-2 servings)

Ingredients:

1 large organic pre-boiled sweet potato, chopped

1 cup pre-cooked organic black lentils

½ cup fresh organic pomegranate seeds (if not in season, replace with grapefruits)

½ cup fresh organic basil, chopped

2-4 organic green onions, chopped

2-4 fresh organic garlic cloves, chopped

3 teaspoons avocado oil

½ cup freshly squeezed organic lemon juice

¼ cup organic apple cider vinegar

½ cup fresh organic cilantro, chopped Himalayan salt and black pepper to taste

Directions:

Put the black lentils, sweet potatoes, green onions and basil in a salad bowl; mix lightly

Season with oil, lemon juice, vinegar, salt and pepper; mix

Toss the pomegranate seeds in and mix

Serve over green salad or as a side dish at room temperature or even cold

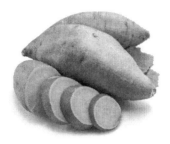

How to Cook the Black Lentils:

Rinse 1 cup of dry black lentils under cold water until water is clear

Transfer lentils to a pot with water (1½ cup of water for every
1 cup of dry lentils)

Bring to a boil, reduce heat and let simmer for about 20-40 minutes or until

lentils are soft (stir occasionally)

Add water if needed but leave partially covered while cooking

Avoid over cooking

Strain water and bring to room temperature before preparing the salad

If you wish, you could substitute some of the water with chicken or

vegetable broth to add more flavor

Cold Tuna and Garbanzo Bean Salad

(1-2 servings)

Ingredients:

½ cup pre-cooked (or canned) garbanzo beans

1 cup water-packed-tuna (or leftover cooked tuna)

½ cup organic carrots cut into strips

½ cup organic cabbage, chopped

½ cup organic green peas

½ cup organic parsley, chopped

¼ cup organic apple cider vinegar

¼ cup freshly squeezed lemon juice

2 medium sized organic garlic cloves, chopped

2 teaspoons avocado oil

Salt and pepper to taste

Directions:

Toss all ingredients into a mid-sized bowl and mix

Spicy Thai Green Bean Salad

(1-2 servings)

Ingredients:

Salad:

1 pound organic pre-steamed or cooked green beans (if not in season, frozen green beans can be used)

¼ raw almonds, chopped

2 organic garlic cloves, chopped

1 teaspoon chili pepper to taste, crushed

½ of an organic onion, chopped

Dressing:

2 teaspoons organic almond butter

2 teaspoons organic rice vinegar

1 teaspoon gluten free soy sauce

1 teaspoon organic honey

1 teaspoon sesame oil

1 teaspoon water

1 teaspoon Himalayan salt

1 teaspoon black pepper

Directions:

Place green beans, almonds, garlic and chili in a mid-sized bowl

Mix all salad dressing ingredients together and set aside

Pour salad dressing on top of the green beans, mix

Sprinkle with chopped onion

Serve at room temperature or cold

Fresh Organic Tabouli Salad

(1-2 servings)

Ingredients:

2 cups pre-cooked organic quinoa

2 fresh organic tomatoes, chopped

2 fresh organic cucumbers, chopped

2 fresh organic red peppers, chopped

10 fresh organic green onions, chopped

2 bunches fresh organic parsley, chopped thinly

1 bunch fresh organic mint, chopped thinly

3 teaspoons organic cold olive oil

2 fresh organic squeezed lemons

1 teaspoon Himalayan salt

3 fresh organic garlic cloves, chopped

Directions

Put all chopped vegetables in a salad bowel

Add the pre-cooked quinoa

Sprinkle with lemon, olive oil & salt

Mix all ingredients, serve cool!

Tabouli is best made as close to serving time as possible

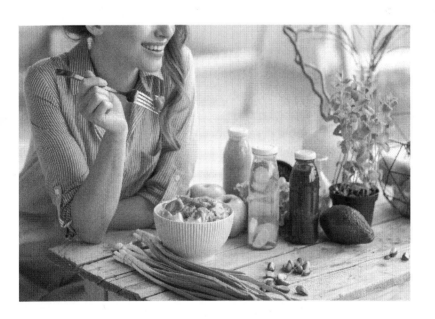

The Great Zucchini!

Zucchini is a great vegetable that you should add to your daily food intake. It has a slightly sweet flavor and ranges in color from dark and bright green to yellow. Zucchinis are delicious cooked, baked, grilled, and even raw. They are rich in minerals and vitamins and will boost your nutrient value. Studies show that consuming zucchinis can support reduction of cholesterol levels, high blood pressure, and blood sugar levels.

By eating 1 cup of zucchini you can get almost 21% of your daily-recommended copper, 10% of magnesium, 12% of vitamin A, 10% of your daily fibers, 19% of manganese, 9% folate. It also contains potassium, an intra-cellular electrolyte mineral, which supports reduction of high blood pressure and heart rate by balancing sodium.

Eating zucchini on a weekly basis will also provide you with 5-7% of the recommended A, B6, B1, B3, B2, C vitamins and 6.3% of the trace mineral zinc that helps regulate blood sugar.

One cup of zucchini is about 35 calories and 4-6 grams of dietary fibers and pectin fibers. Those fibers regulate your insulin and blood sugar levels and support a healthy intestinal mucosa, which aids your digestive tract.

Most importantly, 1 cup of zucchini contains 22mg (24% of our recommended daily intake) of antioxidant vitamin C. Vitamin C dissolves in our body fluids and protects our cells from free radicals that might damage our DNA.

Zucchini Salad
with Basil & Mint

(1-2 servings)

Ingredients:

2-4 fresh organic zucchini, shredded

½ cup of fresh organic basil leaves, chopped

½ cup of fresh organic mint leaves, chopped

2 fresh organic garlic cloves, diced

Sea salt and pepper to taste

2-4 teaspoons of balsamic vinegar

½ cup of fresh organic lemon juice

¼ cup of cold press organic olive oil

Directions

Place the shredded zucchini in a mid-size bowl

Add garlic, mint, and basil leaves

Add olive oil, vinaigrette, and lemon

Season with salt and pepper and mix

All Hail Kale!

Kale is the "Queen of Greens". It's a leafy vegetable in the Brassica family, which also includes broccoli, cauliflower, cabbage, Brussels sprouts, and collard greens. Kale is considered as a super food!

Kale is low in calorie, high in fiber and has zero fat. One cup of kale contains 36 calories, 5 grams of fiber, & 15% of the daily requirement of calcium & vitamin B6 (pyridoxine), 40% of magnesium, 180% of vitamin A, 200% of vitamin C, & 1,020% of vitamin K. It is also a good source of minerals copper, potassium, iron, manganese, and phosphorus.

Kale is a great detox food. It is full of antioxidants, binds bile acids, helps lower blood cholesterol levels and reduce the risk of heart disease.

Here is a great kale salad recipe for you to try!

Kale, Beets and Goat Cheese salad

Ingredients:

1 bunch of organic kale

4-6 pre-cooked, chopped organic beets (red or golden)

50g goat cheese

½ cup of fresh organic lemon

1/2 teaspoon kosher salt

1 tablespoon extra virgin olive oil

Directions

Wash kale, remove leaves and massage them (if needed chopped)

Add the chopped pre-cooked beets

Sprinkle salt

Toss with oil and squeezed lemon juice

Sprinkle with crumbled goat cheese

Mix all ingredients in a large bowl

Serve and enjoy!

Summer Squash Walnut Salad

(1-2 servings)

Ingredients:

4 fresh organic summer squash, chopped

1 cup organic cherry tomatoes

½ cup organic shallot, sliced

¼ cup raw organic walnuts

2 teaspoons cold press olive oil

¼ cup cherry vinegar

2 organic garlic cloves, chopped

1 teaspoon Dijon mustard

Salt and black pepper to taste

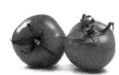

Directions

Mix the chopped summer squash, cherry tomatoes, and sliced shallot in a mid-size bowl

Stir olive oil, vinegar, Dijon mustard, and garlic in a small bowl

Pour the dressing onto the vegetables and mix

Sprinkle with chopped walnuts, salt, and pepper

Super Power Green Salad over Mango and Figs

(1-2 servings)

Ingredients:

4-6 large fresh organic Swiss chard, chopped

1 cup organic spinach, chopped

½ cup organic baby arugula

¼ cup organic alfalfa sprouts

½ cup fresh chives, chopped

¼ cup raw almonds

1 medium fresh mango, peeled and cut into chunks

6 fresh organic figs (black or green), cut into quarters

Salt and pepper to taste

3 teaspoons of cold press olive oil

½ cup of fresh squeezed lemon juice

Directions

In a large bowl, toss together the Swiss chard, spinach, arugula, chives, figs, and mango

Drizzle with olive oil, lemon, and pepper to taste

Add alfalfa sprouts

Sprinkle almonds on top

Ready to serve!

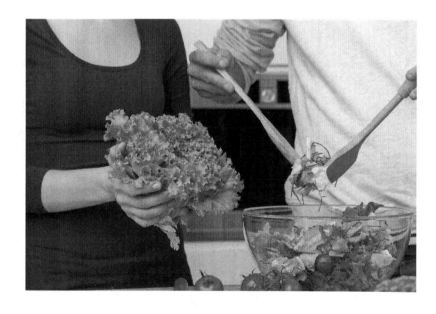

Salad
Dressings

Let's be honest, the dressing makes the salad because it seems every delicious salad depends on the dressing! Most commercial salad dressings contain high-fructose corn syrup and/or different sources of sugar. Some will even have artificial colors or flavors. Creating your own delicious, homemade salad dressings will boost your daily intake of green salads while encouraging you to eat more of these powerful nutritional greens. Go simple, make it easy and try to explore new flavors that will make your culinary experience fun, fulfilling and delicious!

Olive Oil
Vinaigrette Dressing

Ingredients:

3 teaspoon extra virgin olive oil

2 Tablespoons of organic Balsamic vinaigrettes (can be replace with apple cider vinaigrette)

2 Tablespoons of fresh squeezed organic lemon juice

2 cloves fresh organic garlic, chopped

½ teaspoon of sea salt

Directions

Blend all ingredients in a jar.

Adjust flavor if needed (more lemon or salt)

Tahini Lemon Dressing

Ingredients:

2 tablespoons of raw, organic Tahini

½ cup of squeezed fresh organic lemon juice

2 cloves fresh organic garlic, chopped

¼ cup fresh organic parsley, chopped

Kosher salt to taste

1 teaspoon organic paprika powder

¼ to ½ cup of water

Directions

Blend all ingredients in a blender. If the dressing is too thick, add more water. If it is too thin, add more Tahini.

Adjust flavor if needed (more lemon or salt)

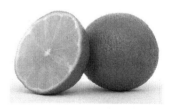

Mustard Flaxseed Oil Vinaigrette Dressing

Ingredients:

3 teaspoons organic flaxseed oil

1 spoonful of organic mustard

2 chopped organic green onion

2 tablespoons of organic Balsamic vinaigrettes (can be replaced with apple cider vinaigrette)

2 tablespoons of fresh organic squeezed lemon juice

2 cloves fresh organic garlic, chopped

½ teaspoon of sea salt

Directions

Blend all ingredients in a jar.

Adjust flavor if needed (more lemon or salt)

Italian Salad Dressing

Ingredients:

3 teaspoons organic sunflower oil

1 spoonful of organic mustard

2 chopped green onion

2 tablespoons of rice vinaigrettes

2 tablespoons of fresh squeezed organic lemon juice

2 cloves fresh organic garlic, chopped

1 teaspoon fresh organic oregano leaves, chopped thinly

½ teaspoon of sea salt

Freshly ground black pepper to taste

Direction:

Blend all ingredients in a jar.

Adjust flavor if needed (more lemon or salt)

Ranch Dressing

Ingredients:

2 tablespoons mayonnaise (* See Note)

Salt and black pepper to taste

2 tablespoons organic cultured buttermilk (** See Note), well-shaken

½ teaspoon rice vinegar

2 cloves fresh organic garlic, chopped

¼ cup of fresh organic chives, chopped

¼ cup of fresh organic mint, chopped

¼ cup of fresh organic parsley, chopped

Direction:

Whisk together all ingredients until you reach the desired consistency. Adjust flavor if needed (more lemon or salt)

Notes:

* If you are looking for a better alternative for mayonnaise, make sure you choose a Gluten-Free, Vegan, Lactose-Free, , Egg-Free, Casein-Free, Soy-Free, No Preservatives, Non-GMO Project Verified mayonnaise. The market is full of options.

** If you can't have dairy, replace dairy with 2 tablespoons of fresh squeezed organic lemon juice

Ginger, Orange Almond Butter Sauce

Ingredients:

1 jar organic almond butter

2 fresh organic oranges, squeezed

2 fresh organic lemons, squeezed

5-10 organic cloves fresh organic garlic, chopped

¼ cup organic cloves fresh organic ginger, chopped

A pinch of salt

Direction:

Blend all ingredients in a jar.

Adjust flavor if needed (more lemon or salt)

Home Made Tahini Paste

Ingredients:

1 cup of raw Tahini (organic sesame paste)

1 cup fresh organic flat leaf parsley, chopped

4-8 fresh organic garlic cloves, chopped

2-3 fresh organic lemons, squeezed

½ cup of water (if needed)

1 teaspoon Kosher salt

1 teaspoon organic paprika

Directions

Blend all ingredients (except the parsley), until you get a soft, smooth and thick consistency (If necessary, add water to thin the consistency)

Add fresh parsley, stir

Transfer tahini to a mason jar, keep stored in the refrigerator for several days

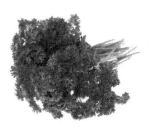

Avocado Dressing

Ingredients:

1-2 ripe avocados

1 garlic clove, chopped

1 teaspoon organic ground cumin

¼ cup fresh organic cilantro, chopped

1-2 fresh organic lemons, squeezed into juice

3 teaspoons water

3 teaspoons extra virgin olive oil

Salt and pepper to taste

Directions:

Cut the avocado in half lengthwise and remove the pit

Scoop out the avocado's flesh and place it in a food processor

Add garlic, cumin and cilantro; mix

Add lemon juice, water and oil (If you like the dressing thinner, add more water)

Season with salt and pepper to taste

Miso Salad Dressing

Ingredients:

1-2 inches of fresh organic ginger, minced

¼ cup white organic miso paste

3 teaspoons rice wine vinegar

1 teaspoon tamari (gluten free soy sauce) or gluten soy sauce

2 teaspoons honey

4 teaspoons sesame oil

Water as needed

Directions:

Place ginger, miso paste, vinegar, tamari and honey in a
food processor; blend until smooth

Slowly add sesame oil into blender and thin dressing to
desired consistency using water

Carrot Vinegar Salad Dressing

Ingredients:

1 cup organic carrot juice

1 teaspoon organic shallots, chopped

1½ teaspoon organic yellow curry powder

1 teaspoon honey

½ cup lemon juice

½ cup extra virgin olive oil Salt and pepper to taste

Directions:

In a small saucepan, heat carrot juice until smooth

In a separate bowl, mix shallot, curry powder, honey and lemon juice

Add carrot juice and whisk together

Add extra virgin olive oil while whisking

Salt and pepper to taste

Hail Caesar Salad Dressing

Ingredients:

½ cup organic grapeseed oil

4-6 organic anchovy fillets (can be replaced with sardines)

2-4 garlic cloves, chopped thinly

2 teaspoons organic Dijon mustard

1 teaspoon Worcestershire sauce (you can choose a gluten free option if needed)

2 yolks from organic eggs

Salt and pepper to taste

1 fresh organic jalapeño, chopped

Directions:

Blend all ingredients until smooth and creamy

Keep in the refrigerator for 2 hours before serving

BlackBerry Vinaigrette

Ingredients:

1 cup fresh organic blackberries*

½ cup avocado oil

½ cup fresh organic orange, peeled

1 inch of fresh organic ginger

½ cup freshly squuezed organic lemon juice
1 teaspoon organic Dijon mustard

Salt and pepper to taste

Directions:

Blend all ingredients in a food processor until you have a
smooth and creamy consistency

* Blackberries can be replaced with blueberries
** If anything is out of season, frozen solutions can be used

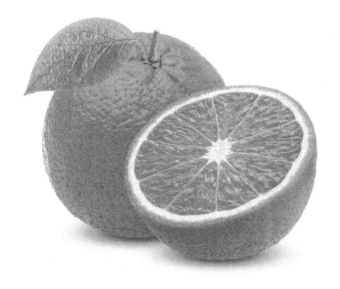

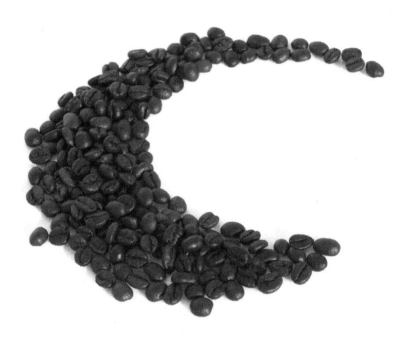

Main
Courses

There are few things more enjoyable than the depth and nutrition made possible by a great main course recipe. With the right recipe, a main course can be filling and delicious without being unhealthy! It does not matter if you are only preparing meals for yourself or for an entire household, there is no doubt you will find recipes you love in this section!

Let's cook!

The "Forbidden Rice"

There is a black rice native to China also known as the "Forbidden Rice". This grain is a great source of the antioxidants flavonoid and anthocyanin as well as dietary fibers, iron and copper. If that's not enough to convince you, this black rice also boasts anti-inflammatory benefits! Incorporating this type of grain into your culinary repertoire will add new flavors and textures while making your dining experience more fun.

The name "Forbidden Rice" was given to this black grain due to the fact common Chinese people were not allowed to grow or eat it. The black rice was served only to the royal and very wealthy people in ancient China. The grains were grown in very limited quantities, monitored and reserved for the highest elite social class.

Half a cup of cooked rice will provide you with approximately 160 calories, 1½ gram of fat, 34 grams of carbohydrates, 2 grams of fiber and 5 grams of protein.

The "Forbidden Rice" is considered to be a gluten free grain. However, if you are pre-diabetic, diabetic, have Celiac disease or have wheat grain sensitivity, then you should consume no more than ½ cup as your serving size.

Now, let's make a great recipe using the "Forbidden Rice".

Forbidden Rice and Beans

(1-4 servings)

Ingredients:

1 cup of pre-cooked Forbidden Rice

1½ cup of water

½ teaspoon Kosher salt

2 teaspoons organic grapeseed oil

½ cup of cooked lima beans (if dry, follow directions)
1 organic white onion, chopped

2 organic tomatoes, chopped

1 fresh organic carrot, cut into strips

1 fresh organic red pepper, cut into strips

1 fresh organic leek, cut into rings

1-2 teaspoons cumin seeds

1½ cup organic, non MSG, gluten free chicken, beef or vegetable broth

½ cup of fresh organic green onions, chopped

¼ cup of organic fresh cilantro, chopped

Directions:

Beans:

Soaking Beans:

½-1 cup dry beans

Soak overnight (8 hours minimum) in cold water

Drain beans, rinse with fresh water

Preparing Beans:

Place beans in a pot and cover with fresh water (about 3-4 cups)

Add chicken, beef or vegetable broth

Cover the soaked beans and boil for 40 minutes

Add vegetables to the broth and beans mixture as if cooking with water

Rice:

Preparing Rice:

Bring 1 cup of rice and 1½ cup of water to a boil in a large saucepan

Lightly season with salt

Cover, reduce heat to low and simmer for about 2-25 minutes or until all
liquid is absorbed and rice is tender

Remove pan from heat and let stand, covered, for 15 minutes

Directions:

Toss rice over cooked beans and vegetables, mix

Sprinkle with fresh green onions and cilantro

Lightly season with salt, if desired

Greek Mediterranean Stuffed Pepper

(4-8 servings)

Ingredients:

10 medium sized organic peppers (green, red or orange)

1 organic onion, chopped

½ cup organic green onions, chopped

2-4 organic tomatoes, chopped

¼ cup organic cilantro, chopped

1½ cup of pre-cooked quinoa

1 cup goat cheese (can be replaced with 1 pound of organic ground beef; if replaced, no need to add shredded chesses)

½ cup shredded chesses 2-4 teaspoons grapeseed oil

1 teaspoon sea salt

2-3 cups water (depending on the pot size)

2-3 teaspoons organic tomato paste

½ teaspoon organic black pepper

1 teaspoon organic cumin seeds

1½ cup of organic, non MSG, gluten free chicken, beef or vegetable broth

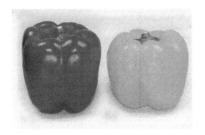

Directions:

Remove and discard the tops, seeds and membranes of the bell peppers, set aside

Filling Preparation:

In a separate bowl, combine pre-cooked quinoa, green onions, cilantro, tomatoes, cheeses, salt, pepper and cumin seeds

Mix all the ingredients together

Stuffed Peppers:

Spoon an equal amount of the mixture into each hollowed pepper, set aside In a large skillet, sauté diced onions with grapeseed oil until tender and brown

Add chicken, beef or vegetable broth with 1 cup of fresh water

Add tomato paste, stir

Arrange peppers in the broth

Bring to boiling point, reduce heat and cook for 20-30 more minutes

Serve over a green salad

Chicken Breast over Mango Salsa

(4-8 servings)

Ingredients:

1 pound boneless, skinless chicken breast cut into 1 inch thick strips

1 teaspoon sesame oil

½ cup tap water

1 organic mango, chopped

¼ cup fresh organic cilantro, chopped

½ cup fresh organic onions, chopped

¼ cup of fresh organic red peppers, chopped

2 fresh organic tomatoes, chopped

½ cup freshly squeezed organic lime juice

1 organic Jalapeño pepper, chopped thinly

2 fresh organic garlic cloves, chopped

¼ teaspoon Himalayan salt

1 teaspoon organic cold pressed avocado oil

½ teaspoon organic cayenne powder

Directions:

Salsa:

Combine chopped mango, onions, tomatoes, peppers, garlic, Jalapeños and cilantro in a bowl

Add avocado oil, lime juice and salt

Mix until well blended

Chicken:

In a pan, sauté chicken breast with sesame oil for 3-7 minutes (medium heat), or until it's golden; season with cayenne

Place chicken breast on a plate and drizzle the mango salsa on top

219

Chicken Breast over Scallions with Ginger and Pineapple Sauce

(2-4 servings)

Ingredients:

1 pound organic boneless, skinless chicken breast cut into

1 inch thick strips

1 teaspoon sesame oil

½ cup water

½ cup fresh organic pineapple, chopped

¼ cup fresh organic onion, chopped

1 tablespoon gluten free organic soy sauce

1 tablespoon rice vinegar

1 teaspoon fresh organic ginger, chopped
2 fresh organic garlic cloves, chopped
¼ cup water

2-4 fresh organic scallions, chopped

Directions:

Combine all ingredients except the scallions, chicken breast and

sesame oil in a bowl; set aside

In a pan, sauté chicken breast with sesame oil for 3-5 minutes
(medium heat)

Add the mixture from the bowl, cook for about 5-7 minutes

Remove from heat and stir in the scallions

Serve over ½ cup of basmati rice or quinoa

Turkey and Bean Burritos

(2-4 servings)

Ingredients:

1 pound organic ground turkey

1 teaspoon sesame oil

1 fresh organic onion, chopped

2-3 fresh organic green onions, chopped

2 fresh organic garlic cloves, chopped

1 cup cooked organic pinto beans

2 fresh organic tomatoes, chopped

2 tablespoons fresh organic avocado, mashed

1 cup fresh organic romaine lettuce, chopped*

½ cup fresh organic cilantro, chopped

1 teaspoon chili powder

1 teaspoon cumin powder

¼ cup water

8 flour tortillas (10 inch diameter)

*Can be replaced with iceberg lettuce or Swiss chard

Directions:

Heat oil in a large skillet and add the onions and garlic, cook for 2 minutes

Add the meat and cook for 4-8 minutes while breaking up the turkey as it cooks

Remove from heat when the mixture turns brownish

Add beans, tomatoes, chili powder, cumin powder and water

Stir and cook over low heat for 10 more minutes

Warm burritos on a pan for 1-2 minutes

Place aside and spread avocado, lettuce, cilantro as well as the turkey and bean mixture

Chicken Lettuce Wraps

(2-4 servings)

Ingredients:

1 pound ground organic chicken

8 fresh organic scallions, chopped

1 fresh organic red bell pepper, chopped

¼ cup organic gluten free, reduced-sodium soy sauce

1 tablespoon fresh organic ginger, chopped

¼ cup water

2 teaspoons sesame oil

1 large head of butter lettuce; washed, dried and separated into leaves

Ingredients for Dipping Sauce:

¼ cup organic gluten free, reduced-sodium soy sauce

¼ cup seasoned rice vinegar

1 tablespoon fresh organic ginger chopped

1 teaspoon sesame oil

2 fresh organic garlic cloves, chopped

Instructions:

Heat oil in large skillet then add onions and garlic

Cook for 2 minutes

Add the meat and cook for 4-8 minutes while breaking up
the chicken as it cooks

Remove from heat when the mixture turns brownish

Add water, soy, scallions, ginger and red peppers, mix until well blended

Cook for a few minutes until the peppers and scallions are soft

In a separate bowl, add all sauce ingredients and mix

Spoon chicken filling onto 1 lettuce leaf and roll

Dip or sprinkle 1 teaspoon of sauce

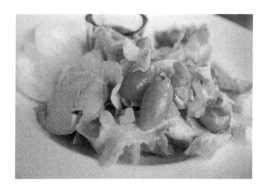

What exactly is Couscous?

Couscous is a Mediterranean product containing gluten and is made from wheat or semolina, which is a type of wheat too. It is very easy to cook and can be used as a side dish. Couscous is a great source of vitamin B6, thiamine, niacin and folate. It supports brain functionality, energy production, the immune system, hormonal balance and is a super source of folate for pregnant women! Couscous also contains the minerals magnesium, choline, calcium, potassium and selenium which regulate metabolism while supporting brain, liver and nerve functions.

A cup of cooked couscous contains about 180 calories, 35 grams of carbohydrates, 2 grams of fiber and 6 grams of protein. If you are cooking it with 1 teaspoon of oil, you will add about 45 more calories to the recipe. The glycemic index for couscous is 65 for 50 grams, however, to be on the safe side, it is recommended to have less than 1 cup of cooked couscous.

Couscous is cooked similarly to rice. For each dry cup of couscous, use 1½ cup of water. Bring water to a boiling point in a mid-sized pot; add salt and 1-2 teaspoons of grapeseed oil or butter if desired. Add 1 cup of dry couscous into the pot, stir and cook for 3-5 minutes. Cover with a lid and let it sit until the water evaporates (about 7 minutes).

If choosing to eat couscous, make sure you consume no more than ½ cup of cooked couscous and try to limit the additional fats (oil and butter) to no more than 2 teaspoons per meal.

Watch out: couscous is NOT a gluten free product!

Here is a great tasting recipe using couscous!

Salmon over Carrots, Cilantro over Couscous on Ghee

(2-4 servings)

Ingredients:

2 organic salmon fillets (¼ pound each)

2 cups pre-cooked organic carrots, chopped into rings

½ cup fresh organic Thai basil, chopped

2-3 fresh organic green onions, chopped

2 fresh organic garlic cloves, chopped

2 teaspoons of organic ghee (*)

½ cup dry cooked couscous (**)

Himalayan salt and black pepper to taste

Directions:

Sprinkle the salmon with salt and pepper

In a pan, sauté salmon fillets with ghee for 5-10 minutes (medium heat)

Flip sides so the salmon will be fully cooked

Transfer to a plate and keep warm

Add onions, garlic and carrots to the warm pan; cook
for 3-5 minutes or until soft

If carrots are not pre-cooked, boil water and add carrots

Cook until they get soft

Rinse water and put aside

Remove from heat

Stir the fresh basil into the carrots mixture

Serve the salmon and vegetables over ½ cup of precooked couscous

Note:

(*) Can be replaced with coconut butter

(**) Can be replaced with quinoa with great results!

Bite Size Chicken Breast with Brussels Sprouts

(4-8 servings)

Ingredients:

1 pound organic chicken breast, cut into bite-size pieces

1 teaspoon sesame oil

2 cups pre-cooked organic Brussels sprouts, chopped into halves

2-3 fresh organic green onions, chopped

1 fresh organic onion, chopped

2 fresh organic garlic cloves, chopped

½ cup freshly squeezed organic lemon juice

¼ cup fresh organic cilantro, chopped

Himalayan salt and black pepper to taste

Directions:

Boil water in a pot

Add Brussels sprouts, cook until they are soft

Rinse with water and put aside

Heat oil in large skillet, sauté onion and garlic for 2 minutes

Add chicken breast, keep cooking for 2 minutes while stirring

Add lemon juice, cilantro, pre-cooked Brussels sprouts and stir

Cook for 5-7 minutes

Season with salt and black pepper

Serve immediately over green salad

Lamb
Fennel Stew

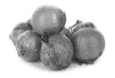

(2-4 servings)

Ingredients:

2 large organic fennel bulbs, chopped

½ cup of dried (or fresh) apricots

½ teaspoon of sea salt

3 pounds of grass fed organic lamb shanks or shoulder blade chops

1 organic onion, chopped

3 organic shallots, chopped

1 cup organic peas (using fresh peas is better,

but frozen ones are acceptable)

1 cup of organic, non MSG mineral broth, vegetable stock or water

Directions:

Preheat oven to 250°F

Line the chopped fennel, onions and shallots in a glass casserole dish

Add lamb, apricots, peas, broth (or water) and salt

Cover and bake for 2½ to 3 hours or until tender

If needed, add ¼ cup water

Serve with steamed vegetables and green salad

Ground Beef and Leek Burgers

(2-4 servings)

Ingredients:

2 large organic leeks, chopped

1/3 cup sesame oil

1 teaspoon of dulse (seaweed)

½ teaspoon of mineral salt

1 pound of grass fed organic beef

Lettuce leaf

1 organic tomato, chopped

1 sliced pickle (optional)

Directions:

Mix the chopped leeks, oil, dulse and salt

Add ground beef and mix

Shape into 3-5 patties, cook on oiled iron skillet over medium heat
for about 15 minutes or until brown

Garnish with lettuce, tomatoes and pickle

Serve with steamed vegetables and green salad

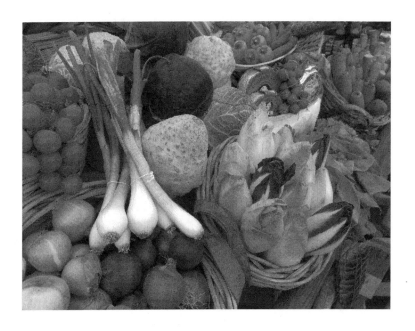

Limonene - The Natural Phytochemical Limonene

Limonene is a super powerful natural chemical found in lemon and orange peels. It is an antioxidant with anti-inflammatory properties which supports our metabolism while blocking cancer cells. This is achieved by shutting down the NF-kappaB gene signals system, which is the central cell regulation for cancer prevention.

As a health compound, it has shown a wonderful ability to help with a variety of health issues including indigestion, acid reflux and sluggish bowels. It is a unique fat cleanser which helps clear cholesterol sludge including in the gall bladder where it can form stones. It also assists with liver detoxification enzymes. In addition, it's calming properties help settle anxiety so it can even be used as a natural sleep aid. It helps reduce appetite and improve metabolism, which assists with healthy weight management. It is also a superior nutrient for breast cancer prevention!

You should use organic lemon or organic orange peels if you are planning to cook with it in your dishes. It's always a good idea to avoid pesticides or other chemicals in your food whenever possible. When you see commercial foods with the label "d-limonene", you should know it is a lab made commercial extraction. If you can't find organic lemons or oranges, soak the fruits in fresh water, then rinse (there's still no guarantee the pesticides and chemicals will not be in your food).

Consider using lemon in your cooking as often as you can. It can be added to savory or sweet dishes and it is also a key ingredient in homemade salad dressings. A mid-sized lemon has numerous nutritional benefits and only 14 calories, so why not use it?

As you have already seen, I love using lemons and lemon juice in my recipes! That being said, here is yet another scrumptious recipe featuring the magical lemon touch!

Chicken Drumsticks over Green Olive, Lemon, Paprika & Turmeric

(4-8 servings)

Ingredients:

6-10 organic chicken drumsticks

2 organic lemons with the peel, chopped

2 organic carrots, peeled and cut into strips

2-3 organic white onions, chopped

2 teaspoons organic paprika powder

2-4 teaspoons organic turmeric powder

½ cup green olives, pickled and pitted

1 teaspoon black pepper

1-3 cups water

1 cup organic chicken broth, MSG free

Directions:

In a large pot, bring chicken broth and water to a boil then reduce heat

Add chicken drumsticks to the pot

Add onions, chopped lemons, carrots, green olives, paprika, turmeric and black pepper

Stir all ingredients and cook for about 30-40 minutes

Serve over ½ cup of cooked basmati rice, quinoa or millet

Orange Chicken Burgers with Fresh Tomatoes & Pickles

(2-4 servings)

Ingredients:

40 ounces (1kg) organic ground chicken (*)

1 organic egg, beaten

2 organic white onions, chopped

2 organic tomatoes, chopped

1 small organic red pepper, chopped

1 organic orange, chopped

1 teaspoon grapeseed oil

1 teaspoon Himalayan salt

1 teaspoon black pepper

¼ teaspoon cumin seeds

1-2 teaspoons organic mustard

¼ cup fresh organic Swiss chard, chopped

1 teaspoon organic apple cider vinegar

2-3 dill pickles and/or pickled Jalapeño peppers

If using home pan for cooking, add 2 teaspoon of vegetable oil

2 slices of bread (gluten free bread is the best option for your health) (**)

Directions:

Swiss chard: drizzle with 1 teaspoon of organic apple cider vinegar and a pinch of salt, set aside

In a medium bowl, combine all ingredients until you reach a unified consistency

Use your hands to shape the burger sized patties and place them on a plate

Barbecue burger patties over medium heat

Spread organic mustard on bread slices

Top with freshly sliced tomatoes, Swiss chard, pickles and/or some pickled Jalapeño peppers

Notes:

(*) Ground Chicken breast can be replaced with Turkey, Lamb or Ground Beef

(**) if gluten free, you can replace the bread slices with iceberg lettuce to make a wrap burger, it's delicious and very healthy!

Salmon with Mustard, Chia Seeds and Ginger

(2-4 servings)

Ingredients:

1½ pound fresh wild salmon fillet, cut into 4-8 pieces

1 fresh organic onion, chopped

1-2 fresh garlic cloves, chopped

¼ cup organic, gluten free soy sauce

¼ cup fresh organic cilantro, chopped

¼ cup fresh organic ginger, chopped

2 fresh lemons, squeezed into juice

2 teaspoons organic Dijon mustard

2 teaspoons chia seeds

½ cup chicken or vegetable broth, MSG free

½ cup water

Salt and black pepper to taste

Directions:

In a large stainless steel skillet, bring water, soy sauce
and broth to a boil then reduce heat

Add onion, cilantro and ginger; cook for 4-6 minutes

Rub salmon fillet with Dijon mustard, chia seeds, salt and black pepper

Place salmon fillet in hot skillet and cook for 5 minutes on each side
(it cooks quickly so don't overcook it)

Top the serving fillet with lemon juice and garlic

Serve with green salad and 1 cup of cooked quinoa

Italian Style Veal with Spaghetti Squash

(2-4 servings)

Ingredients:

16 oz organic veal breast

3-6 fresh organic garlic cloves, chopped

4 fresh organic tomatoes, chopped

¼ cup fresh organic oregano leaves, chopped (if out of season, use dried leaves) 1 cup fresh organic parsley, chopped

4 cups winter Spaghetti squash, baked

1 teaspoon sesame oil

1 teaspoon black pepper

½ cup water

Directions:

Heat oil in a large pot over medium heat

Season veal with black pepper and oregano on both sides

Carefully add veal to the hot pan, cook until both sides are brown

Reduce heat; add garlic, tomatoes and parsley

Add water and cook for about 45 minutes

Serve over cooked Spaghetti squash

The Classic Roasted Chicken

(2-4 servings)

Ingredients:
6 organic chicken drumsticks

3 organic shallots, chopped

3 organic potatoes, chopped

3 organic carrots, chopped

2 organic onions, chopped

1 teaspoon paprika

2 organic garlic cloves, chopped

2 organic sprig rosemary bunches

Salt and pepper to taste

1 cup water

Directions:
Preheat oven to 400°F

Place chicken pieces in a bowl; sprinkle with salt, pepper, garlic,
shallot, paprika and rosemary

Rub the seasonings onto the chicken

Set the chicken in a glass baking pan over the chopped potatoes, carrots
and onion

Add water and roast in the oven for 30-40 minutes or until skin is brown

Add water if needed

Halibut with Dijon and Almonds

(2-4 servings)

Ingredients:

½ fillet Halibut (Wild, Atlantic or Pacific are better than farmed)

2 teaspoons organic Dijon

2 teaspoons raw almonds, chopped

2 organic garlic cloves, chopped

Salt and pepper to taste

1-2 teaspoons coconut oil

Directions:

Preheat oven to 350°F

Lightly grease baking sheet with coconut oil

Lay fish in the pan and spread Dijon over it

Sprinkle with chopped almonds and garlic

Bake for 12-15 minutes or until fish flakes easily with a fork

Spread coconut oil just before serving for final moisture touch

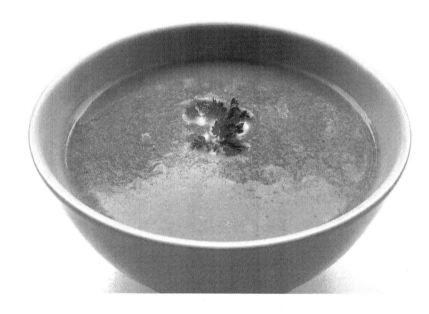

Soups

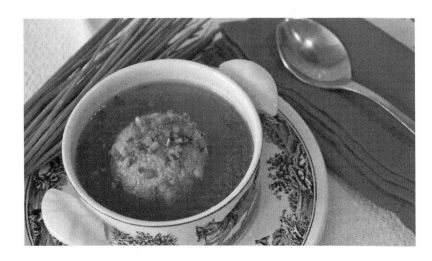

There are few things more soothing than warm or even hot soup when the weather turns brisk. Making soup can be a labor of love, but when the fragrant aroma of a simmering soup fills the household air, good vibes are spread throughout! Maybe a little hunger too! No need to worry though, with these recipes there will be enough soup for everybody!

Winter Roots Vegetable Soup

Ingredients:

3-5 organic carrots, peeled and cut

2-3 organic zucchini, peeled and cut

2 organic potatoes, peeled and cut

1 organic sweet potato, peeled and cut

2-3 organic Jerusalem artichokes, peeled and cut

2 organic white onions, chopped

3 organic garlic cloves, chopped

2-3 organic bay leaves

6-8 organic whole allspice cloves

6-8 whole black peppercorns

1 organic fennel tube, sliced or cut

1 organic celery root, peeled or cut into cubes

1 organic parsley root, peeled and cut

1 organic tomato, cut into cubes

1 organic red pepper, cut roughly

½ cup of porcini mushrooms

½ bunch of fresh organic parsley leaves

½ bunch of fresh organic dill leaves

2-3 stalks of organic celery, cut

½ cup organic lemon juice (optional)

Tap water or bottled water to cover the vegetables
(amount depends on pot size)

1 cup organic mineral broth (optional)

2-3 teaspoons of Turmeric

2-3 teaspoons organic ginger, peeled and cut (add more ginger for
stronger flavor)

Directions:

Put all herbs in the bottom of a large pot (parsley, dill,
celery, bay leaves and fennel)
Add cut vegetables on top
Add mushrooms, tomatoes and red peppers
Add spices, turmeric, allspice cloves, black pepper,
garlic, lemon juice and ginger
Add water (to cover the vegetables) and bring to a boil
Lower heat to let simmer and keep cooking for 1½ hour
Serve with fresh lemon

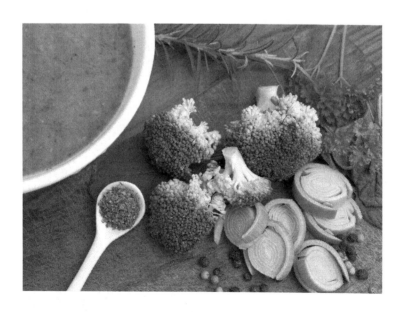

Think Spices!

Spices are the pearls of Mother Nature as well as the variety of life! They will add color and an interesting twist to raw food or any dish for that matter. If that's not enough, spices also benefit your health!

Incorporating spices in your diet will support your immune system tremendously. Most spices have antibacterial, antifungal as well as anti-inflammatory mineral and trace mineral properties which strengthen your immune system. Spices are created from roots, seeds, fruits or bark. The quality of the spice's source matters because it's the soil the plant is growing in which drives the nutritional value of the spices up. Go organic and non-GMO to make sure you purchase high quality spices.

General Guidelines: Spices should be used in very small amounts. Generally, you should use between ¼ to 1 teaspoon per dish. Always start with a smaller amount of spices, then add more if needed. It's better to add spices in the beginning of the cooking process to allow flavors to blend and absorb. On the other hand, herbs should be added at the end of the process.

Store spices in a covered container and place it in a dark, dry place (not close to source of heat such as a stove or microwave because it will damage the quality of the spices you are using).

Buy in small amounts and refresh your stock every six months.

Freshness depends on the smell. The stronger the smell is, the fresher your spice is. Simply smell your spices to check freshness!

Shelf Life: read the label date. Most sales and deals are close to expiration dates.

Make sure you buy a product that has at least 1 year until its expiration date.

Cardamom is a super antioxidant, anti-inflammatory and anticancer spice. It has a strong flavor. Cardamom supports the digestion system, especially if one is struggling with candida, gut dysbiosis, SIBO, IBS or leaky gut. It's also helpful for gas, bloating, heartburn or constipation as well. Due to the potent diuretic and fibers in cardamom, it also lowers high blood pressure and prevents blood clots by preventing platelet aggregation.

Use whole pod or ground (no need to crack, unless it is specified in the recipe) if possible. You should know that whole pods have a much stronger taste. The pods need to be heated before use to release their essential oils. Another option is to sauté the spices in oil and then add them to your recipe.

Cumin is a great spice which supports the digestive system due to its powerful essential oils; cuminaldehyde which activates our salivary glands and thymol which stimulates bile as well as digestive enzymes in the GI track. Cumin has anti-fungal, antimicrobial and anticarcinogenic enzymes. It is also a great source of iron containing 66mg in every 100 grams of cumin. Obviously no one eats 100 grams of cumin daily! However, using cumin on a weekly basis helps maintain healthy red blood cells carrying oxygen to cells. This process helps prevent anemia. Cumin also regulates sleep, strengthens the immune system and improves memory!

Cumin is one of the basic ingredients in some of the most popular spices; curry and chili powder. Using either of those two spice blends will provide you with some of the health benefits of cumin as well.

Cumin can be added to meat, eggs, beans, lentils, vegetables and grains. It provides a strong, warm and earthy aroma to any dish. Surprisingly, it can also be used to make tea. Cumin can be used as a whole seed or in powder form.

Caraway also supports the digestive system, especially those who suffer from heart-burn, bloating, gas or loss of appetite. It relieves stomach and intestines spasms as well. Caraway has anti-fungal, antimicrobial, anti-infection and anticarcinogenic enzymes. It supports a healthy heart rate while lowering both high blood pressure and high cholesterol levels.

The essential oil Galactogogue found in caraway seeds can increase milk production for lactating mothers. The quantity and the quality of the milk will improve as you introduce more caraway in your diet. For a quick and easy way to get more caraway, I recommend mixing caraway seeds with honey and spreading it on a slice of bread.

Use caraway to improve the taste of your food or salad dressings by blending it with other spices and herbs to enrich your dishes. It can be used in baked goods or with meat, cheese, sauerkraut and pickles.

Turmeric – Curcumin is the active component in turmeric and is the most studied spice on earth. Turmeric is a super antioxidant, anti-inflammatory, antibacterial, antifungus and anti cancer spice. Turmeric truly is a super spice!

Turmeric supports a healthy gut and is helpful for those who have heartburn, stomach pain, diarrhea, gas or bloating. It supports a healthy gallbladder, liver and kidney detoxification. It reduces infections and joint inflammation (arthritis), skin problems as well as colds. Studies show that curcumin blocks NF-kB, a protein molecule that interferes with the DNA nuclei and cytokins production. It also activates the genes related to shutting down inflammation pathways.

The taste is a bit bitter, therefore I recommend a maximum of ½ to 1 teaspoon a day. Turmeric turns the color of anything it touches to a strong, dark yellow; this includes your skin, pots and pans! You can cook the root or use fresh organic powder. You can boil, sauté or cook turmeric. You can use it over vegetables, fruits, fish, meat and even coffee too. It's a wonderful culinary addition to any dish you make and delivers tremendous health benefits to you as well!

Nutmeg is another great spice, but is generally not used in the western culinary kitchen with the exception of holiday seasons. Nutmeg supports our digestive system by regulating the peristaltic motion in the muscles of the intestines. It improves brain function as it contains the essential oils myristicin and macelignan. It also supports liver detoxification, boosts skin health, strengthens the immune system and improves blood circulation. Not to mention, it also contains fibers, vitamins and minerals such as vitamin B6, copper, folate, thiamin and manganese. These all play an important role in our health!

It has a sweet and warm flavor that goes great with desserts, soups, sauces as well as Mediterranean and Indian meat dishes.

You can use the whole or ground powder form in your cooking. The whole seed form has a much stronger flavor compared to the ground form. Just like any potent spice, you should use small amounts of it frequently. I recommend using nutmeg once or twice per week.

Saffron is definitely the most expensive spice. It's exotic, powerful and tasty; you should also include it in your diet.

Saffron is a great source of magnesium, manganese, vitamin C, iron, potassium and B6. These all play a key role in balancing our mood, repairing or forming cells, regulating blood sugar, supporting carbohydrate metabolism and absorbing calcium. Saffron contains 4 carotenoid antioxidants: zeaxanthin, lycopene as well as alpha and beta carotene. These keep free radicals in check.

Before adding saffron to your dish, you will want to soak it in warm water for 1 minute so the flavor essence is released into the liquid. Then, transfer the liquid into the dish you are cooking. Always use a very small amount of saffron in your cooking, a pinch should be enough. It's a great addition to fish, rice, quinoa, soup, bread or baked goods.

Speaking of soup, let's make one together that contains these phenomenal spices!

The Six Powerful
Spices Soup

Ingredients:

3-4 pounds organic chicken, cut into 6-8 pieces

Tap water or bottled water to cover ingredients (amount depends on pot size)

3 large organic onions, peeled and cut into quarters

4-6 organic carrots, cut into rings

5-8 stalks of fresh organic celery, cut

3 potatoes, cut into half rings across with a thickness of 2 inches

1 cup organic cauliflower, chopped

2 organic leeks, cut into rings

1-2 tablespoons of six powerful spice blend (see recipe next page)

1 large bunch of organic cilantro, chopped

Salt and black pepper, freshly ground

Directions:

Put all ingredients in a large pot

Add water

Bring to a boil and reduce heat, cook for 1 -1½ hours

Serve with fresh cilantro

Note: for stronger flavor, add organic non MSG chicken broth

The Six Powerful Spices Blend

Ingredients:

10 whole cardamom seeds

3-4 clove grains

½ cup organic cumin powder

1 teaspoon caraway

½ cup black pepper

1 teaspoon of organic Turmeric, powder

1/2 teaspoon of organic Nutmeg, powder

1/2 teaspoon of organic Saffron, powder

Directions:

Mix all ingredients and grains together

Note: this mixture of spices can sit for 6 months and can be used for other dishes as well

You need 1-2 tablespoons of the mixture for a soup

Know Your Mushrooms!

Mushrooms belong to the fungi kingdom and they are considered a super food! Most mushrooms provide us with iron, niacin, potassium, copper, selenium and vitamin D. They also contain many antioxidants such as ergothioneine, a naturally occurring antioxidant. They provide us with amino acids that contain sulfur, which provides DNA cellular protection against free radical damage but mainly helps lower blood pressure. The antioxidant ergosterol turns into vitamin D when exposed to ultraviolet light but they also contain lovastatin, which has been shown to significantly reduce cholesterol levels in rats. Another antioxidant found in mushrooms is known as pantothenic acid, it helps support the nervous system as well as hormone production.

There are only 20-28 calories in every ½ cup of mushrooms. This makes them a great addition to your nutritional daily intake, especially if you want to lose weight! Studies proved that consuming 1 cup of mushrooms every day over a 12 month span will reduce your weight by 7 pounds!

You must be careful to use certified organic mushrooms because mushrooms absorb any pollutants or chemicals from the soil and environment they grow in.

You can eat mushrooms raw, cooked, steamed or baked. Add them to any dish you're creating and they will lend their earthy flavor to your dish.

Many mushroom recipes suggest adding butter, ghee or lard to sweeten the pot.

If you are dairy free, coconut butter or any other liquid oil can be a great substitute.

If you're using dry mushrooms, you want to rinse and soak them for 20-30 minutes in water before cooking them. Then, squeeze and dry them. You can even use the soaked water in the dish you're making to get more nutritional benefits.

Although I never freeze my mushrooms, you could consider doing so. You can store them in a sealed container for up to 1-2 months.

Beware! Some wild mushrooms can be toxic and harmful. Make sure you choose edible ones. If you have a slight doubt, don't eat them!

Don't just stick to popular mushrooms such as white mushrooms, Portobello and Crimini. Get out of your comfort zone and try some different varieties such as Maitake, Shiitake, Reishi, Oyster mushrooms, King Trumpet, Enoki, Hen of the Wood as well as White and Brown Beech! You'll be glad you did!

Ok, let's make that wild mushroom soup now!

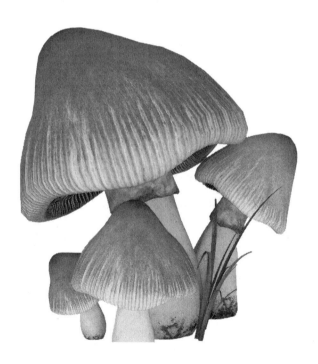

Wild Mushrooms Soup

Ingredients:

1½ cup organic Portobello mushrooms, sliced

1½ cup organic Oyster mushrooms, sliced

2 cups organic Beech mushrooms

1½ cup organic Shiitake mushrooms, sliced

1½ cup organic Crimini (or Porcini) mushrooms

2 organic potatoes, diced

2 organic carrots, cut into rings

5 garlic cloves, minced

½ cup dry white wine

2 cups vegetable stock, non MSG

2-3 teaspoons organic butter

1 cup of heavy organic cream

Salt and pepper to taste

2 tablespoons fresh organic oregano, chopped

Tap water or bottled water to cover ingredients

(amount depends on pot size)

Directions:

Clean mushrooms and cut into bite-sized pieces, set aside

Boil water and then add vegetables

Add cream, wine and butter

Boil for the second time and then reduce heat

Add onions, potatoes and carrots; cook for 10-15 minutes

Add mushrooms and cook for another 20-30 minutes

Add oregano and/or thyme

Season with salt and pepper to taste

Sprinkle fresh oregano on each dish

Note:

Skip the wine if you can't have sugar or alcohol

For stronger flavor, add 1-2 sprigs of fresh thyme, divided

If the soup is too thick, you can add water to thin it

Turkey Meat Balls, Kale & Spinach Soup

Ingredients:

2 organic white onions, chopped

2-3 organic carrots, chopped

1 organic zucchini, chopped

2 stalks of organic celery, chopped

2 cups fresh organic spinach

2 cups fresh organic kale, chopped

½ teaspoon lemon zest

1 pound organic ground turkey breast

¼ to ½ cup of precooked quinoa

½ cup fresh organic parsley, chopped

½ cup fresh organic basil, chopped 4-6 fresh organic garlic cloves, minced

2-3 cups organic chicken broth, non MSG

Salt and pepper to taste

1 organic beaten egg

Tap water or bottled water to cover ingredients (amount depends on pot size)

Directions:

Turkey meatballs:

Combine ground turkey, quinoa, basil, parsley, garlic and egg

Mix together until well combined

Shape into meatballs

Put aside

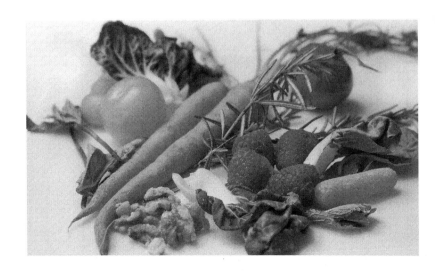

Soup:
Boil water and add the shaped meatballs
Cook for 15-20 minutes then reduce heat
Add vegetables, white onions, carrots, zucchini and celery
Add salt, black pepper and chicken broth; cook for 20-30 minutes
Add the spinach and kale, cook for 10 more minutes

Serve with fresh lemon and garlic

Chicken Meatballs, Leek, Carrots and Italian Parsley Soup

Ingredients:

2 organic white onions, chopped

2 organic leeks, chopped

6-8 organic carrots, chopped

1-2 cups fresh organic Italian parsley, chopped

1 pound organic ground chicken breast

¼ to ½ cup of pre-cooked brown rice

½ cup fresh organic dill, chopped

4-6 fresh organic garlic cloves, minced

2-3 cups organic chicken broth, non MSG

Salt and pepper to taste

2 teaspoons organic sweet paprika

1 teaspoon organic turmeric

1 organic beaten egg

Tap water or bottled water to cover ingredients
(amount depends on pot size)

Directions:

Chicken meatballs:

Combine ground chicken, rice, dill, garlic and egg

Mix together until well combined

Shape into meatballs

Put aside

Soup:

Boil water and chicken broth

Add the meatballs and cook for 15-20 minutes then reduce heat

Add vegetables, white onions, leeks and carrots

Add salt, black pepper, paprika, turmeric and cook for 20-30 minutes

Add parsley and cook for 10 more minutes

Serve with fresh garlic

Note: you can puree soup (vegetables and meatballs) in a blender or with an immersion blender for a thicker result

Chicken Soup with Lemon Grass, Bock Choy and Celery

Ingredients:

1 whole organic skinless chicken divided into 6-8 pieces

3-5 organic carrots, peeled and cut into rings

2-3 organic bok choy, chopped

1 large organic white onion, chopped

2 large organic leeks, chopped

1 organic celery root, peeled and cut into quarters

1 organic parsley root, peeled and quartered

1 organic turnip, peeled and divided

1 organic kohlrabi, peeled and halved

3 large sticks of organic lemon grass cut into smaller sticks
(you can break them into halves)

½ cup fresh organic ginger root, peeled and freshly sliced

1 large bunch of organic parsley

1 large bunch of organic cilantro

4-6 organic garlic cloves, minced

Salt and black pepper to taste

2-3 cups organic chicken broth, non MSG

2 tablespoons organic gluten-free soy sauce

½ cup fresh organic sliced green onions

Tap water or bottled water to cover ingredients
(amount depends on pot size)

Directions:

Boil water with the chicken broth

Add chicken pieces and cook for 15-20 minutes then reduce heat

Add lemon grass, soy sauce and vegetables; cook for 30-45 minutes
or until chicken is soft

Add herbs: cilantro, parsley, ginger and garlic; cook for 10 more minutes
(add jalapeño chilies if desired)

Add salt and black pepper to taste

Sprinkle with green onions before serving

Note:

Lemon grass

Rinse lemon grass in water

Cut each stalk into 3-4 inches

Lightly crush lemon grass to get the flavors out If you like more spice, you can add 1 organic jalapeño chili at the herb stage You can also add ½ cup of rice noodles or dry egg noodles to a bowl of soup to enrich the dish

Minestrone Soup

Ingredients:

2 tablespoons organic cold pressed olive oil

1 organic white onion, chopped

3-6 organic garlic cloves, finely sliced or minced

2-4 organic carrots, peeled and cut into rings

2-3 organic zucchinis, cut into cubes

2-3 organic potatoes, cut into cubes

2-3 stalks of fresh organic celery, diced

1 cup pre-soaked lima beans (see directions)

4 organic tomatoes, cut into small cubes

2 tablespoons organic tomato paste

1 bunch of fresh organic basil, chopped

Salt and black pepper to taste

1-2 fresh sprigs of organic oregano leaves

1 cup short pasta, cooked "al dente" (if gluten free, choose either gluten free option of pasta or buckwheat grains)

1 cup organic chicken or vegetable broth, non MSG

Tap water or bottled water to cover ingredients
(amount depends on pot size)

Directions:

Boil water with chicken broth then reduce heat

Add lima beans and root vegetables then cook for 30-45 minutes

Add pasta, cook for 10 minutes

Add basil and tomato paste, stir; cook for 10 more minutes

Add salt, black pepper and oregano, stir; remove from heat

Add olive oil and stir

Garnish with fresh organic basil

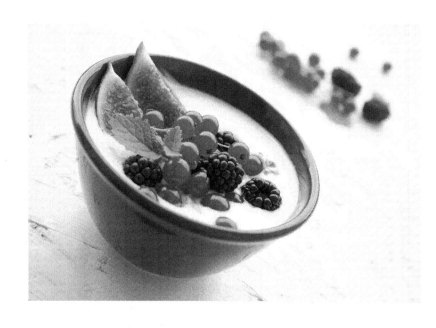

Dessert and Baking

Did you know the best part of the meal doesn't have to be the most dangerous to your health? There are healthier ways to make desserts and sweet treats without sacrificing flavor! It's so important to understand ingredients, especially when it comes to so called "sugar substitutes" which are really just clever names used for sugar itself. The first question we should really ask is whether or not each ingredient listed on prepackaged sweets and treats is even real food! The best way to know for sure is to just make your own at home!

Enough sweet talk, here is why it's called home sweet home!

Medjool Dates with Pistachio and Coconut

Ingredients:

10-15 organic Medjool Dates

2-4 teaspoons of organic pistachios

¼ cup organic Tahini (sesame seed paste)

Shredded, unsweetened coconut for sprinkling over the top

Directions:

Slice each date halfway through the center

Remove the pit and open the date up slightly, without separating the halves

Insert 1-2 pistachios

Drizzle Tahini over the dates

Sprinkle shredded coconut over the top

Refrigerate the dates to keep fresh

Classic Oat Bran Muffins

Ingredients:

¾ cup almond milk

1 tablespoon freshly squeezed organic lemon juice

½ cup organic oat bran

1 ¾ cup of whole oats

1 teaspoon aluminum free baking powder

¼ teaspoon sea salt

¼ cup raw almonds, chopped

¾ cup cottage cheese; use organic apple sauce or banana if you are
sensitive to dairy

Organic grapeseed oil, spray

Directions:

Preheat oven to 400°F

Spray muffin cups with oil and set aside

Combine almond milk with lemon juice in a cup and set
aside for 10 minuets

Combine dry ingredients in a large bowl

Add the almond milk mixture, cottage cheese (or applesauce/banana) and
mix gently until completely moistened

Spoon into prepared muffin cups until ¼ full

Bake for 20-30 minutes or until lightly brown

Cool down for at least 10 minutes before removing from pan

Apple & Banana Muffins

Ingredients:

½ cup organic almond flour 4 large eggs

2 medium apples; peeled, cored and chopped

2 medium bananas

¼ cup almond oil

1½ teaspoon baking powder

2 teaspoons ground cinnamon

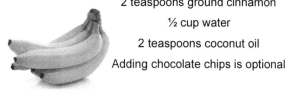

½ cup water

2 teaspoons coconut oil

Adding chocolate chips is optional

Directions:

Preheat to 350°F, spray muffin cups with oil and set aside

In a large bowl, mix fruits (use a potato masher)

Add flour, baking powder, cinnamon, eggs, oils and water; mix

Fill prepared muffin cups halfway with mixture

Baked for 15 minutes (check, bake for 5 more minutes if needed)

Let cool before removing from muffin tin

keep refrigerated and the muffins will last about 5 days

Morning Vegetable Muffins

Ingredients:

¼ cup tomatoes, chopped

¼ cup mushrooms, chopped

¼ cup mixed greens: spinach, parsley, basil and green onions; chopped

¼ cup shredded sheep cheese

¼ cup goat cheese

Pinch of cumin seeds, salt and pepper

6 eggs, beaten

2 tablespoons almond flour

1 teaspoon aluminum free baking powder

Directions:

Preheat to 350°F, spray muffin cups with oil and set aside

In a large bowl, mix chopped vegetables

Add flour, baking powder, cumin seeds, cheese and eggs; mix

Fill prepared muffin cups halfway with mixture

Bake for 15 minutes (check, bake for 5 more minutes if needed)

Let cool before removing from muffin tin

These are great for breakfast!

Cold Almond Milk Pudding

Ingredients:

2 cups unsweetened almond milk

1 teaspoon organic vanilla extract

½ cup organic almond flour

¼ cup organic hemp seeds

1-2 teaspoons organic cinnamon powder

Directions:

Heat the almond milk and stir, reduce heat

Add the almond flower, stir; cook for 3 more minutes, remove from heat

Add the hemp seeds, stir

Pour into a pudding mold or individual serving dishes; It's easier to unmold if they've been lightly sprayed or wiped with a little oil

Sprinkle a pinch of cinnamon on top of each serving

Cover with plastic wrap and refrigerate until set

Blueberry Amaranth Porridge

Ingredients:

1½ cup Amaranth (uncooked)

2½ cups water

2½ cups almond milk

2 tablespoons butter

⅓ cup coconut butter (substitute almond, cashew or peanut butter)

½ cup chopped apple (or mango, banana, raspberries, etc.)

1 teaspoon chia seeds (substitute hemp or poppy seeds)

1 tablespoon maple syrup (or less)

Cinnamon or coca can be added to enrich flavor if desired

Directions:

Combine amaranth, water, almond milk and coconut butter on a small pan

Bring to a boil, reduce heat; keep cooking about 15-20 minutes

Add chia seeds and maple syrup, mix

Add the blueberries and apples

Transfer into a jar

Serve immediately or eat chilled (refrigerate overnight, keeps up to 3 days)

Flax Seeds
and Walnut Balls

Ingredients:

1 cup raw organic walnuts

½ cup organic flax seeds 3 dry, dioxin free apricots

3 organic dry seeded dates

½ cup organic coconut spread (Wilderness Family) 1 teaspoon organic vanilla extract

Directions:

Process all ingredients in a food processor until it's combined

Roll into small balls (about 1 inch in diameter)

Place in a container and refrigerate

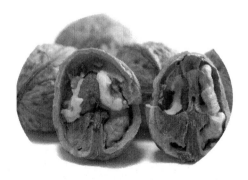

Tahini Cookies

Ingredients:

½ cup organic butter/Ghee

½ cup raw organic sugar

½ teaspoon pure vanilla extract

2 cups organic tahini (sesame seed paste)

3/5 cup Farro flour

2 teaspoons baking powder

1 organic egg

¼ cup carob chocolate chips or whole almonds

Directions:

Preheat oven to 350°F

Line a baking sheet with parchment paper

Mix butter (or ghee) with sugar until fluffy

Add egg, vanilla and Tahini; mix until well combined

In a separate bowl, sift together the flour and baking powder;
stir into butter mixture

With wet hands, roll a ball with about 1 tablespoon of the mix,

place on the baking sheet

Brush cookies with scrambled egg

Put one almond or carob chocolate chip in center of each cookie
and push it down

Bake in preheated oven until they turn golden brown, about 15 minutes.

Thyme, Sesame, Salt and Pepper Crackers

Ingredients:

1 cup white sesame seeds

1 cup black sesame seeds

¼ cup poppy seeds

½ cup rice flour (can be replaced with almond or coconut flour)

2 teaspoons dry organic thyme

½ teaspoon sea salt

½ teaspoon black peeper

½ teaspoon cumin seeds

½ to 1 cup of water

¼-½ cup of sesame oil

Directions:

Place flour, sesame seeds (white and black), thyme, poppy, cumin, salt and pepper in mid-size bowl; mix (optional: you can use oregano and rosemary)

Add water and oil, mix until soft and a bit sticky (if too dry, add more water 1 teaspoon at a time; mix should not be too loose)

Place mixture over a piece of parchment paper - flat, thin and equal using tablespoon

Bake at 365°F for 15-25 minutes (or until edges turn brown)

Allow to cool for a few minutes, cut baked dough into

squares using pizza cutter or knife

Keep cooling the square crackers for 30 more minutes before transferring to container

Crackers last for 2-3 weeks

Gluten Free, Egg Free, and Dairy Free Pizza Crust

Ingredients:

For the crust:

1 cup brown rice flour (can be replaced with quinoa or almond flour)

1 cup potato or tapioca starch

1 teaspoon Xanthan Gum

2 tablespoons aluminum free baking powder

¾ teaspoon sea salt

1 teaspoon brown sugar

¼ cup avocado oil

¾ cup almond milk or water

For the toppings:

½ cup tomatoes, chopped

¼ cup mushrooms, chopped

¼ cup red peppers, chopped

¼ cup olives

1 teaspoon dried oregano

3-6 fresh basil leaves

¼ cup goat or sheep cheese (shredded or cubed)

Directions:

Preheat oven to 400°F

Mix all dry ingredients in a bowl: flour, tapioca starch, Xanthan Gum, baking powder, sea salt and brown sugar

Add oil and almond milk to dry ingredients and stir, make sure all dry ingredients are absorbed completely

Grease a round pizza pan

Place dough on the pan; bake for 5-7 minutes

Remove from the oven and top with cheese, tomatoes, peppers, olives, mushrooms, oregano and basil leaves; place back inside oven and bake for 15-25 more minutes Allow a few minutes to cool, slice and serve!

Making granola bars is super easy and so much healthier as well as more delicious than prepackaged bars. You can control the ingredients thus providing you and your child a healthy snack without chemicals or preservatives. Not to mention, you'll avoid high fructose corn syrup and the "good source of whole grain" or whatever the food company mean by that! This is exactly why I designed a great granola bar recipe to make at home. Perfect as a light breakfast or snack combined with yogurt, honey, fresh strawberries or bananas.

Granola Bars

Ingredients:

1 cup almond butter

1½ cup peanut butter

1½ teaspoon vanilla extract

1½ cup brown sugar

1 cup maple syrup or agave syrup

5 cups quick cooking oats (organic)

1 cup coconut

2 teaspoons hemp seeds

2 teaspoons chia seeds

1 cup sunflower seeds

1 cup sesame seeds

1 cup carob chocolate chips (optional)

½ cup raisins

Directions:

Using a skillet, lightly toast the coconut, hemp, chia,
sunflower and sesame seeds; set aside
In a large mixing bowl, combine the butter, peanut butter, vanilla and sugar
Add the syrup then mix in the oats, raisins, chocolate chips and the
toasted ingredients Press into a greased 12x18 inch cookie
sheet and bake at 350°F for about 20 minutes or until golden brown
Let cool slightly before cutting into squares while still warm

REFERENCES

The Gluten-Free Weight Loss Connection

1. Dickey, W., & Kearney, N. (2006). Overweight in celiac disease: Prevalence, clinical characteristics, and effect of a gluten-free diet. *The American journal of gastroenterology, 101*(10), 2356-2359.

2. Gaesser, G. A., & Angadi, S. S. (2012). Gluten-free diet: Imprudent dietary advice for the general population? *Journal of the Academy of Nutrition and Dietetics, 112*(9), 1330-1333.

3. Hafekost, K., Lawrence, D., Mitrou, F., O'Sullivan, T. A., & Zubrick, S. R. (2013). Tackling overweight and obesity: does the public health message match the science? *BMC medicine, 11*(1), 1.

4. Kabbani, T. A., Goldberg, A., Kelly, C. P., Pallav, K., Tariq, S., Peer, A., & Leffler, D. A. (2012). Body mass index and the risk of obesity in coeliac disease treated with the gluten-free diet. *Alimentary pharmacology & therapeutics, 35*(6), 723-729.

5. Mann, T., Tomiyama, A. J., Westling, E., Lew, A. M., Samuels, B., & Chatman, J. (2007). Medicare's search for effective obesity treatments: diets are not the answer. *American Psychologist, 62*(3), 220.

6. Marcason, W. (2011). Is there evidence to support the claim that a gluten-free diet should be used for weight loss? *Journal of the American Dietetic Association, 111*(11), 1786.

7. Miller, W. C., (1999). How effective are traditional dietary and exercise interventions for weight loss? *Medicine and Science in Sports and Exercise, 31*(8), 1129-1134.

8. Sonti, R., & Green, P. H. (2012). Celiac disease: Obesity in celiac

disease. *Nature Reviews Gastroenterology and Hepatology*, *9*(5), 247-248.

9. Ukkola A, Mäki M, Kurppa K, Collin P, Huhtala H, Kekkonen L, Kaukinen K. (2012), Changes in body mass index on a gluten-free diet in coeliac disease: a nationwide study, Eur J Intern Med. Jun;23(4):384-8.

Losing control

1. FACSI, A. B. M. C. F., Dashti, H. M., Mathew, T. C., & Hussein, T. (2004). Long-term effects of a ketogenic diet in obese patients.

2. Gaesser, G. A., & Angadi, S. S. (2012). Gluten-free diet: Imprudent dietary advice for the general population? *Journal of the Academy of Nutrition and Dietetics*, *112*(9), 1330-1333.

3. Hursting, S. D., Dunlap, S. M., Ford, N. A., Hursting, M. J., & Lashinger, L. M. (2013). Calorie restriction and cancer prevention: a mechanistic perspective. *Cancer & metabolism*, *1*(1),

4. Mann, T., Tomiyama, A. J., Westling, E., Lew, A. M., Samuels, B., & Chatman, J. (2007). Medicare's search for effective obesity treatments: diets are not the answer. *American Psychologist*, *62*(3), 220.

5. Rosenbaum, M., Hirsch, J., Gallagher, D. A., & Leibel, R. L. (2008). Long-term persistence of adaptive thermogenesis in subjects who have maintained a reduced body weight. *The American journal of clinical nutrition*, *88*(4), 906-912.

6. Westman, E. C., Feinman, R. D., Mavropoulos, J. C., Vernon, M. C., Volek, J. S., Wortman, J. A., & Phinney, S. D. (2007). Low-carbohydrate nutrition and metabolism. *The American journal of clinical nutrition*, *86*(2), 276-284.

7. Researchers at Washington University. Retrieved from http://umm.edu/health/medical/reports/articles/weight-control-and-diet

Low Carbohydrate Diet vs. Gluten-Free Diet

1. Higdon, H. (2006). "Fiber Fact Sheet." The Linus Pauling Institute Micronutrient Information Center. International Food information Council (IFIC).

2. Kreitzman, S. N., Coxon, A. Y., & Szaz, K. F. (1992). Glycogen storage: illusions of easy weight loss, excessive weight regain, and distortions in estimates of body composition. *The American journal of clinical nutrition, 56*(1), 292S-293S.

3. Phinney, S. D., Bistrian, B. R., Evans, W. J., Gervino, E., & Blackburn, G. L. (1983). The human metabolic response to chronic ketosis without caloric restriction: preservation of submaximal exercise capability with reduced carbohydrate oxidation. *Metabolism, 32*(8), 769-776.

4. McGuire, S. (2010). US Department of Agriculture and US Department of Health and Human Services, Dietary Guidelines for Americans. Washington, DC: US Government Printing Office, January 2011. *Advances in Nutrition: An International Review Journal, 2*(3), 293-294.

5. Moshfegh, A., Goldman, J., & Cleveland, L. (2010). What we eat in America, NHANES 2001-2002: usual nutrient intakes from food compared to dietary reference intakes. *US Department of Agriculture, Agricultural Research Service, 9.*

6. Simopoulos, A. P. (2001). The Mediterranean diets: what is so special about the diet of Greece? The scientific evidence. *The Journal of nutrition, 131*(11), 3065S-3073S.

7. Sparks, L. M., Xie, H., Koza, R. A., Mynatt, R., Hulver, M. W., Bray, G. A., & Smith, S. R. (2005). A high-fat diet coordinately downregulates genes required for mitochondrial oxidative phosphorylation in skeletal muscle. *Diabetes, 54*(7), 1926-1933.

8. Weiss, R., Dufour, S., Taksali, S. E., Tamborlane, W. V., Petersen, K. F., Bonadonna, R. C., & Savoye, M. (2003). Prediabetes in obese youth: a syndrome of impaired glucose tolerance, severe insulin resistance, and altered myocellular and abdominal fat partitioning. *The Lancet, 362*(9388), 951-957.

9. Wilson, D. H., Bogacz, J. P., Forsythe, C. M., Turk, P. J., Lane, T. L., Gates, R. C., & Brandt, D. R. (1993). Fully automated assay of glycohemoglobin with the Abbott IMx analyzer: novel approaches for separation and detection. *Clinical chemistry, 39*(10), 2090-2097. http://www.webmd.com/diet/compare-dietary-fibers

The Gluten-free Diet

1. Afify, A. E. M. M., El-Beltagi, H. S., El-Salam, S. M. A., & Omran, A. A. (2011). Bioavailability of iron, zinc, phytate and phytase activity during soaking and germination of white sorghum varieties. *Plos one, 6*(10), e25512.

2. Annette K Taylor, MS, PhD, CGC, Benjamin Lebwohl, MD, MS, Cara L Snyder, MS, CGC, and Peter HR Green, MD (2016). Synonyms: œliac Disease, Celiac Sprue, Nontropical Sprue, Gluten-Sensitive Enteropathy, Pagon RA, Adam MP, Ardinger HH, et al., editors.

3. Aziz, I., Hadjivassiliou, M., & Sanders, D. S. (2014). Self-reported gluten sensitivity: an international concept in need of consensus? *The American journal of gastroenterology, 109*(9), 1498.

4. Barlow, J., Johnson, J. A. P., & Scofield, L. (2007). Early Life Exposure to the Phytoestrogen Genistein and Breast Cancer Risk in Later Years. *Breast Cancer & the Environment Research Centers Fact Sheet on the Phytoestrogen Genistein. University of California San Francisco*, 47-55.

5. Baudon, J. J., Boulesteix, J., Lagardere, B., & Fontaine, J. L. (1976). Acute villous atrophy due to intolerance to soy bean protein. *Archives françaises de pédiatrie, 33*(2), and 153.

6. Bock, S. A., & Atkins, F. M. (1990). Patterns of food hypersensitivity during sixteen years of double-blind, placebo-controlled food challenges. *The Journal of pediatrics, 117*(4), 561-567.

7. Bohn, L., Meyer, A. S., & Rasmussen, S. K. (2008). Phytate: impact on environment and human nutrition. A challenge for molecular breeding. *Journal of Zhejiang University Science B, 9*(3), 165-191.

8. Buscarini, E., Conte, D., Cannizzaro, R., Bazzoli, F., De Boni, M., Delle Fave, G., & Spolaore, P. (2014). White paper of Italian Gastroenterology: delivery of services for digestive diseases in Italy: weaknesses and strengths. *Digestive and Liver Disease, 46*(7), 579-589.

9. Camarca, A., Anderson, R. P., Picascia S, Bassi V, Facchiano, A., Pisapia L., & Troncone, R. (2016). Intestinal T cell responses to gluten peptides are largely heterogeneous: implications for a peptide-

based therapy in celiac disease. *The Journal of Immunology*, *182*(7), 4158-4166.

10. Catassi, C., Bai, J. C., Bonaz, B., Bouma, G., Calabrò, A., Carroccio, A., & Francavilla, R. (2013). Non-celiac gluten sensitivity: the new frontier of gluten related disorders. *Nutrients*, *5*(10), 3839-3853.

11. Cheng, G., Wilczek, B., Warner, M., Gustafsson, J. Å. & Landgren, B. M. (2007). Isoflavone treatment for acute menopausal symptoms. *Menopause*, *14*(3), 468-473.

12. Cianferoni, A. (2016). Wheat allergy: diagnosis and management. *Journal of asthma and allergy*, *9*, 13.

13. Dall, M., Calloe, K., Haupt-Jorgensen, M., Larsen, J., Schmitt, N., Josefsen, K., & Buschard, K. (2013). Gliadin Fragments and a Specific Gliadin 33-mer Peptide Close K ATP Channels and Induce Insulin Secretion in INS-1E Cells and Rat Islets of Langerhans. *PloS one*, *8*(6), e66474.

14. Dalla Pellegrina, C., Perbellini, O., Scupoli, M. T., Tomelleri, C., Zanetti, C., Zoccatelli, G., & Chignola, R. (2009). Effects of wheat germ agglutinin on human gastrointestinal epithelium: insights from an experimental model of immune/epithelial cell interaction. *Toxicology and applied pharmacology*, *237*(2), 146-153.

15. European Journal of Inflammation. 2008 Jan-Apr;6(1):1721-1727

16. Fric, P., Gabrovska, D., & Nevoral, J. (2011). Celiac disease, gluten-free diet, and oats. *Nutrition reviews*, *69*(2), 107-115.

17. Gibson, P. R., & Shepherd, S. J. (2010). Evidence-based dietary management of functional gastrointestinal symptoms: The FODMAP approach. *Journal of gastroenterology and hepatology*, *25*(2), 252-258.

18. Gibson, P. R., & Shepherd, S. J. (2012). Food choice as a key management strategy for functional gastrointestinal symptoms. *The American journal of gastroenterology*, *107*(5), 657-666.

19. Global Gluten-Free Market to Reach 6.2 Billion by 2018. (2013). *Food Export*. Retrieved 5 February 2017, from https://www.foodexport. org/docs/default-source/newsletters/global_food_marketer/2013/ novemberdecember2013globalfoodmarketer.pdf?sfvrsn=2

20. Gluten-Free Labeling of Foods. (2013). *FDA*. Retrieved 5 February 2017, from https://www.fda.gov/food/guidanceregulation/ guidancedocumentsregulatoryinformation/allergens/ucm362510. htm

21. Gupta, R. K., Gangoliya, S. S., & Singh, N. K. (2015). Reduction of phytic acid and enhancement of bioavailable micronutrients in food grains. *Journal of food science and technology, 52*(2), 676-684.

22. Hershko, C., & Patz, J. (2008). Ironing out the mechanism of anemia in celiac disease. *Haematologica, 93*(12), 1761-1765.

23. Howdle, P. D. (2006). Gliadin, glutenin or both? The search for the Holy Grail in coeliac disease. *European journal of gastroenterology & hepatology, 18*(7), 703-706.

24. Huebner, F. R., Lieberman, K. W., Rubino, R. P., & Wall, J. S. (1984). Demonstration of high opioid-like activity in isolated peptides from wheat gluten hydrolysates. *Peptides, 5*(6), 1139-1147.

25. Hurrell, R. F. (2003). Influence of vegetable protein sources on trace element and mineral bioavailability. *The Journal of nutrition, 133*(9), 2973S-2977S.

26. Hurrell, R. F., Juillerat, M. A., Reddy, M. B., Lynch, S. R., Dassenko, S. A., & Cook, J. D. (1992). Soy protein, phytate, and iron absorption in humans. *The American journal of clinical nutrition, 56*(3), 573-578.

27. Inomata, N. (2009). Wheat allergy. *Current opinion in allergy and clinical immunology, 9*(3), 238-243.

28. Jackson, J. R., Eaton, W. W., Cascella, N. G., Fasano, A., & Kelly, D. L. (2012). Neurologic and psychiatric manifestations of celiac disease and gluten sensitivity. *Psychiatric Quarterly, 83*(1), 91-102.

29. Krüger, M., Shehata, A. A., Schrödl, W., & Rodloff, A. (2013) Glyphosate suppresses the antagonistic effect of Enterococcus spp. on Clostridium botulinum. *Anaerobe, 20*, 74-78.

30. Kristjánsson, G., Venge P., & Hällgren, R. (2007). Mucosal reactivity to cow's milk protein in coeliac disease. *Clinical & Experimental Immunology, 147*(3), 449-455.

31. Leduc, V., Moneret-Vautrin, D. A., Guerin, L., Morisset, M., & Kanny, G. (2003). Anaphylaxis to wheat isolates: immunochemical study of a case proved by means of double-blind, placebo-controlled food challenge. *Journal of allergy and clinical immunology*, *111*(4), 897-899.

32. Li, F. N., Li, L. L., Yang, H. S., Yuan, X. X., Zhang, B., Geng, M. M., ... & Yin, Y. L. (2011). Regulation of soy isoflavones on weight gain and fat percentage: evaluation in a Chinese Guangxi minipig model. *Animal*, *5*(12), 1903-1908.

33. Lie, B. A., Akselsen, H. E., Joner, G., Dahl-Jørgensen, K., Rønningen, K. S., Thorsby, E., & Undlien, D. E. (1997). HLA associations in insulin-dependent diabetes mellitus: no independent association to particular DP genes. *Human immunology*, *55*(2), 170-175.

34. Ludvigsson, J. F., Leffler, D. A., Bai, J. C., Biagi, F., Fasano, A., Green, P. H., & Lundin, K. E. A. (2013). The Oslo definitions for coeliac disease and related terms. *Gut*, *62*(1), 43-52.

35. Maglio, M., Mazzarella, G., Barone, M. V., Gianfrani, C., Pogna, N., Gazza, L., & Miele, E. (2011). Immunogenicity of two oat varieties, in relation to their safety for celiac patients. *Scandinavian journal of gastroenterology*, *46*(10), 1194-1205.

36. Marsh, M. N. (1992). Gluten, major histocompatibility complex, and the small intestine: a molecular and immunobiologic approach to the spectrum of gluten sensitivity ('celiac sprue'). *Gastroenterology*, *102*(1), 330-354.

37. Matsuo, H., Morita, E., Tatham, A. S., Morimoto, K., Horikawa, T., Osuna, H., & Dekio, S. (2004). Identification of the IgE-binding epitope in ω-5 gliadin, a major allergen in wheat-dependent exercise-induced anaphylaxis. *Journal of Biological Chemistry*, *279*(13), 12135-12140.

38. Mesnage, R., Clair, E., Gress, S., Then, C., Székács, A., & Séralini, G. E. (2013). Cytotoxicity on human cells of Cry1Ab and Cry1Ac Bt insecticidal toxins alone or with a glyphosate-based herbicide. *Journal of Applied Toxicology*, *33*(7), 695-699.

39. Mishkind, M., Keegstra, K., & Palevitz, B. A. (1980). Distribution of wheat germ agglutinin in young wheat plants. *Plant physiology*, *66*(5), 950-955.

40. Murray, K., Wilkinson-Smith, V., Hoad, C., Costigan, C., Cox, E., Lam, C., & Spiller, R. C. (2014). Differential effects of FODMAPs (fermentable oligo-, di-, mono-saccharides and polyols) on small and large intestinal contents in healthy subjects shown by MRI. *The American journal of gastroenterology, 109*(1), 110-119.

41. Padgette, S. R., Taylor, N. B., Nida, D. L., & Bailey, M. R. (1996). The composition of glyphosate-tolerant soybean seeds is equivalent to that of conventional soybeans. *The Journal of Nutrition, 126*(3), 702.

42. Pagon, R. A., Bird, T. D., & Dolan, C. R. Seattle (WA): University of Washington, Seattle; 1993. *Available at: External link: http:// www. ncbi. nlm. nih. Gov./books/NBK1157.*

43. Perkkiö, M., Savilahti, E., & Kuitunen, P. (1981). Morphometric and immunohistochemical study of jejunal biopsies from children with intestinal soy allergy. *European journal of pediatrics, 137*(1), 63-69.

44. Pisapia, L., Camarca, A., Picascia, S., Bassi, V., Barba, P., Del Pozzo, G., & Gianfrani, C. (2016). HLA-DQ2. 5 genes associated with celiac disease risk are preferentially expressed with respect to non-predisposing HLA genes: Implication for anti-gluten T cell response. *Journal of autoimmunity, 70*, 63-72.

45. Pruimboom, L., & de Punder, K. (2015). The opioid effects of gluten exorphins: asymptomatic celiac disease. *Journal of Health, Population and Nutrition, 33*(1), 24.

46. Raboy, V., & Dickinson, D. B. (1984). Effect of phosphorus and zinc nutrition on soybean seed phytic acid and zinc. *Plant physiology, 75*(4), 1094-1098.

47. Real, A., Comino, I., de Lorenzo, L., Merchán, F., Gil-Humanes, J., Giménez, M. J., & Barro, F. (2012). Molecular and immunological characterization of gluten proteins isolated from oat cultivars that differ in toxicity for celiac disease. *PLOS one, 7*(12), e48365.

48. Rubio-Tapia, A., & Murray, J. A. (2010). Celiac disease. *Current opinion in gastroenterology, 26*(2), 116.

49. Rubio-Tapia, A., Hill, I. D., Kelly, C. P., Calderwood, A. H., & Murray, J. A. (2013). ACG clinical guidelines: diagnosis and management of

celiac disease. *The American journal of gastroenterology, 108*(5), 656-676.

50. Sampson, H. A. (1999). Food allergy. Part 1: immunopathogenesis and clinical disorders. *Journal of Allergy and Clinical Immunology, 103*(5), 717-728.

51. Sampson, H. A., Mendelson, L., & Rosen, J. P. (1992). Fatal and near-fatal anaphylactic reactions to food in children and adolescents. *New England Journal of Medicine, 327*(6), 380-384.

52. Samsel, A., & Seneff, S. (2013). Glyphosate, pathways to modern diseases II: Celiac sprue and gluten intolerance. *Interdisciplinary toxicology, 6*(4), 159-184.

53. Sapone, A., Bai, J. C., Ciacci, C., Dolinsek, J., Green, P. H., Hadjivassiliou, M., & Ullrich, R. (2012). Spectrum of gluten-related disorders: consensus on new nomenclature and classification. *BMC medicine, 10*(1), 13. No 57

54. Saturni, L., Ferretti, G., & Bacchetti, T. (2010). The gluten-free diet: safety and nutritional quality. *Nutrients, 2*(1), 16-34.

55. Senapati, T., Mukerjee, A. K., & Ghosh, A. R. (2009). Observations on the effect of glyphosate based herbicide on ultra-structure (SEM) and enzymatic activity in different regions of alimentary canal and gill of Channa punctatus (Bloch). *Journal of Crop and Weed, 5*(1), 236-245.

56. Shehata, A. A., Schrödl, W., Aldin, A. A., Hafez, H. M., & Krüger, M. (2013). The effect of glyphosate on potential pathogens and beneficial members of poultry microbiota in vitro. *Current microbiology, 66*(4), 350-358.

57. Shepherd, S. J., Parker, F. C., Muir, J. G., & Gibson, P. R. (2008). Dietary triggers of abdominal symptoms in patients with irritable bowel syndrome: randomized placebo-controlled evidence. *Clinical Gastroenterology and Hepatology, 6*(7), 765-771.

58. Silano, M., Pozo, E. P., Uberti, F., Manferdelli, S., Del Pinto, T., Felli, C., & Restani, P. (2014). Diversity of oat varieties in eliciting the early inflammatory events in celiac disease. *European journal of nutrition, 53*(5), 1177-1186.

59. Sollid, L. M., Markussen, G., Ek, J., Gjerde, H., Vartdal, F., &

Thorsby, E. (1989). Evidence for a primary association of celiac disease to a particular HLA-DQ alpha/beta heterodimer. *Journal of Experimental Medicine, 169*(1), 345-350.

60. Tandon, N., Zhang, L., & Weetman, A. P. (1991). HLA associations with Hashimoto's thyroiditis. *Clinical endocrinology, 34*(5), 383-386.

61. Tang, D., Dong, Y., Ren, H., Li, L., & He, C. (2014). A review of phytochemistry, metabolite changes, and medicinal uses of the common food mung bean and its sprouts (Vigna radiata). *Chemistry Central Journal, 8*(1), 4.

62. Torre, M., Rodriguez, A. R., & Saura-Calixto, F. (1991). Effects of dietary fiber and phytic acid on mineral availability. *Critical Reviews in Food Science & Nutrition, 30*(1), 1-22.

63. Vader, W., Kooy, Y., van Veelen, P., de Ru, A., Harris, D., Benckhuijsen, W., ... & Koning, F. (2002). The gluten response in children with celiac disease is directed toward multiple gliadin and glutenin peptides. *Gastroenterology, 122*(7), 1729-1737.

64. Valladares, L., Garrido, A., & Sierralta, W. (2012). Soy isoflavones and human health: breast cancer and puberty timing. *Revista medica de Chile, 140*(4), 512-516.

65. Van de Wal, Y., Kooy, Y. M., van Veelen, P., Vader, W., August, S. A., Drijfhout, J. W., & Koning, F. (1999). Glutenin is involved in the gluten-driven mucosal T cell response. *European journal of immunology, 29*(10), 3133-3139.

66. Van den Broeck, H. C., de Jong, H. C., Salentijn, E. M., Dekking, L., Bosch, D., Hamer, R. J., & Smulders, M. J. (2010). Presence of celiac disease epitopes in modern and old hexaploid wheat varieties: wheat breeding may have contributed to increased prevalence of celiac disease. *Theoretical and Applied Genetics, 121*(8), 1527-1539.

67. Velasquez, M. T., & Bhathena, S. J. (2007). Role of dietary soy protein in obesity. *Int J Med Sci, 4*(2), 72-82.

68. Veraverbeke, W. S., & Delcour, J. A. (2002). Wheat protein composition and properties of wheat glutenin in relation to breadmaking functionality. *Critical Reviews in Food Science and Nutrition, 42*(3), 179-208.

69. Verdu, E. F., Armstrong, D., & Murray, J. A. (2009). Between celiac disease and irritable bowel syndrome: the "no man's land" of gluten sensitivity. *The American journal of gastroenterology, 104*(6), 1587-1594.

70. Vojdani, A. (2009). Detection of IgE, IgG, IgA and IgM antibodies against raw and processed food antigens. *Nutrition & metabolism, 6*(1), 22. No 71

71. Volta, U., Bardella, M. T., Calabrò, A., Troncone, R., & Corazza, G. R. (2014). An Italian prospective multicenter survey on patients suspected of having non-celiac gluten sensitivity. *BMC medicine, 12*(1), 85.

72. http://www.csaceliacs.org/gluten_free_whole_grains_health_fact_sheet.jsp

73. http://www.ncbi.nlm.nih.gov/pmc/articles/PMC3681969/

74. http://www.fda.gov/NewsEvents/Newsroom/PressAnnouncements/ucm363474.htm

75. https://www.ncbi.nlm.nih.gov/books/NBK1727/

76. http://www.fda.gov/Food/ResourcesForYou/Consumers/ucm079311.htm

77. http://www.uchospitals.edu/pdf/uch_007937.pdf

78. https://www.ebi.ac.uk/interpro/entry/IPR001419

79. Hill ID, Dirks MH, Liptak GS, et al., (2005). Guideline for the diagnosis and treatment of celiac disease in children: recommendations of the North American Society for Pediatric Gastroenterology, Hepatology, and Nutrition. J Pediatr Gastroenterol Nutr. 40:1-19.

80. Rostom A, Murray JA, Kagnoff MF (2006). American Gastroenterological Association (AGA) Institute technical review on the diagnosis and management of celiac disease. Gastroenterology. 131:1981-2002

Nutrient Imbalances

1. Aasheim, E. T., Hofsø, D., Hjelmesæth, J., Birkeland, K. I., & Bøhmer, T. (2008). Vitamin status in morbidly obese patients: a cross-sectional study. *The American journal of clinical nutrition*, *87*(2), 362-369

2. Actor, J. K., Hwang, S. A., & Kruzel, M. L. (2009). Lactoferrin as a natural immune modulator. *Current pharmaceutical design*, *15*(17), 1956-1973.

3. Adams, J. S., & Hewison, M. (2010). Update in vitamin D. *The Journal of Clinical Endocrinology & Metabolism*, *95*(2), 471-478.

4. Alavian, S. M., Motlagh, M. E., Ardalan, G., Motaghian, M., Davarpanah, A. H., & Kelishadi, R. (2008). Hypertriglyceridemic waist phenotype and associated lifestyle factors in a national population of youths: CASPIAN Study. *Journal of tropical pediatrics*, *54*(3), 169-177.

5. Allen, L. H. (2008). Causes of vitamin B12 and folate deficiency. *Food and nutrition bulletin*, *29*(2_suppl1), S20-S34.

6. Bernstein, C. N., Leslie, W. D., & Leboff, M. S. (2003). AGA technical review on osteoporosis in gastrointestinal diseases. *Gastroenterology*, *124*(3), 795-841.

7. Blackburn, P., Lemieux, I., Alméras, N., Bergeron, J., Côté, M., Tremblay, A., & Després, J. P. (2009). The hypertriglyceridemic waist phenotype versus the National Cholesterol Education Program–Adult Treatment Panel III and International Diabetes Federation clinical criteria to identify high-risk men with an altered cardiometabolic risk profile. *Metabolism*, *58*(8), 1123-1130.

8. Blackburn, P., Lemieux, I., Lamarche, B., Bergeron, J., Perron, P., Tremblay, G., & Després, J. P. (2012). Hypertriglyceridemic waist: a simple clinical phenotype associated with coronary artery disease in women. *Metabolism*, *61*(1), 56-64.

9. Bode, S., & Gudmand-Høyer, E. (1996). Symptoms and haematologic features in consecutive adult coeliac patients. *Scandinavian journal of gastroenterology*, *31*(1), 54-60.

10. Bourre, J. M. (2006). Effects of nutrients (in food) on the structure and function of the nervous system: update on dietary requirements

for brain. Part 1: micronutrients. *Journal of Nutrition Health and Aging*, *10*(5), 377.

11. Cannizzaro, R., Da Ponte, A., Tabuso, M., Mazzucato, M., De Re, V., Caggiari, L., & Canzonieri, V. (2014). Improving detection of celiac disease patients: a prospective study in iron-deficient blood donors without anemia in north Italy. *European journal of gastroenterology & hepatology*, *26*(7), 721-724.

12. Carlsson, A. C., Risérus, U., & Ärnlöv, J. (2014). Hypertriglyceridemic waist phenotype is associated with decreased insulin sensitivity and incident diabetes in elderly men. *Obesity*, *22*(2), 526-529.

13. Corazza, G. R., Di Sario, A., Cecchetti, L., Tarozzi, C., Corrao, G., Bernardi, M., & Gasbarrini, G. (1995). Bone mass and metabolism in patients with celiac disease. *Gastroenterology*, *109*(1), 122-128.

14. Dahele, A., & Ghosh, S. (2001). Vitamin B12 deficiency in untreated celiac disease. *The American journal of gastroenterology*, *96*(3), 745-750.

15. Damms-Machado, A., Weser, G., & Bischoff, S. C. (2012). Micronutrient deficiency in obese subjects undergoing low calorie diet. *Nutrition journal*, *11*(1), 34.

16. Darling, A. L., Millward, D. J., Torgerson, D. J., Hewitt, C. E., & Lanham-New, S. A. (2009). Dietary protein and bone health: a systematic review and meta-analysis. *The American journal of clinical nutrition*, ajcn-27799.

17. Del Valle, H. B., Yaktine, A. L., Taylor, C. L., & Ross, A. C. (Eds.). (2011). Dietary reference intakes for calcium and vitamin D. *National Academies Press*.

18. DeVault K. R., & Talley, N. J. (2009). Insights into the future of gastric acid suppression. *Nature Reviews Gastroenterology and Hepatology*, *6*(9), 524-532.

19. Fernández-Bañares, F., Monzón, H., & Forné, M. (2009). A short review of malabsorption and anemia. *World J Gastroenterol*, *15*(37), 4644-52.

20. Gasche, C., Lomer, M. C. E., Cavill, I., & Weiss, G. (2004). Iron, Anaemia, and inflammatory bowel diseases. *Gut*, *53*(8), 1190-1197.

21. Greger, J. L., Baligar, P., Abernathy, R. P., Bennett, O. A., & Peterson, T. (1978). Calcium, magnesium, phosphorus, copper, and manganese balance in adolescent females. *The American journal of clinical nutrition, 31*(1), 117-121.

22. Halfdanarson, T. R., Litzow, M. R., & Murray, J. A. (2006). Hematologic manifestations of celiac disease. *Blood, 109*(2), 412-421.

23. Hallert, C., Grant, C., Grehn, S., Grännö, C., Hultén, S., Midhagen, G., & Valdimarsson, T. (2002). Evidence of poor vitamin status in coeliac patients on a gluten-free diet for 10 years. *Alimentary pharmacology & therapeutics, 16*(7), 1333-1339.

24. Kaidar-Person, O., Person, B., Szomstein, S., & Rosenthal, R. J. (2008). Nutritional deficiencies in morbidly obese patients: a new form of malnutrition? *Obesity surgery, 18*(8), 1028-1034.

25. Keast, D. R., Fulgoni, V. L., Nicklas, T. A., & O'Neil, C. E. (2009). Food sources of energy and nutrients among children in the United States: *U.S. Department of Agriculture/Economic Research Service Nutrients, 5*(1), 283-301.

26. Kemppainen, T. (1997). Oat Meal as a Component of a Glutenfree Diet, Nutrient Intakes, Nutritional Status and Osteopenia in Coeliac Patients. *University of Kuopio.*

27. Kemppainen, T., Uusitupa, M., Janatuinen, E., Järvinen, R., Julkunen, R., & Pikkarainen, P. (1995). Intakes of nutrients and nutritional status in coeliac patients. *Scandinavian journal of gastroenterology, 30*(6), 575-579.

28. Kerns, J. C., Arundel, C., & Chawla, L. S. (2015). Thiamin deficiency in people with obesity. *Advances in Nutrition: An International Review Journal, 6*(2), 147-153.

29. Kerstetter, J. E., Looker, A. C., & Insogna, K. L. (2000). Low dietary protein and low bone density. *Calcified tissue international, 66*(4), and 313-313.

30. Kinsey, L., Burden, S. T., & Bannerman, E. (2008). A dietary survey to determine if patients with coeliac disease are meeting current healthy eating guidelines and how their diet compares to that of the British general population. *European journal of clinical nutrition, 62*(11), 1333-1342.

31. Kocuvan Mijatov, M. A., & Mičetić-Turk, D. (2016). Dietary Intake In Adult Female Coeliac Disease Patients In Slovenia. *Slovenian Journal of Public Health*, *55*(2), 96-103.

32. Kong, J., Zhang, Z., Musch, M. W., Ning, G., Sun, J., Hart, J., & Li, Y. C. (2008). Novel role of the vitamin D receptor in maintaining the integrity of the intestinal mucosal barrier. *American Journal of Physiology-Gastrointestinal and Liver Physiology*, *294*(1), G208-G216.

33. Kraus, J., & Schneider, R. (1979). Pernicious anemia caused by Crohn's disease of the stomach. *American Journal of Gastroenterology*, *71*(2).

34. LeBlanc, E. S., Rizzo, J. H., Pedula, K. L., Ensrud, K. E., Cauley, J., Hochberg, M., & Hillier, for the Study of Osteoporotic Fractures, T. A. (2012). Associations between 25-hydroxyvitamin D and weight gain in elderly women. *Journal of women's health*, *21*(10), 1066-1073.

35. Leite Vieira, D. C., Tajra, V., da Cunha, D., lopes de Farias, D., de Oliveira, A., gomes Teixeira, T., ... & Prestes, J. (2013). Decreased functional capacity and muscle strength in elderly women with metabolic syndrome. *Clinical interventions in aging*, *8*, 1377-1386.

36. Lindner, A., Charra, B., Sherrard, D. J., & Scribner, B. H. (1974). Low vitamin D and narcolepsy and cataplexy, Sleep. *New England Journal of Medicine*, *290*(13), 697-701.

37. Lodato F, Azzaroli F, Turco L, et al. (2010). Association of long-term proton pump inhibitor therapy with bone fractures and effects on absorption of calcium, vitamin B12, iron, and magnesium. *Current gastroenterology reports*, *12*(6), 448-457.

38. Lönnerdal, B. (2009). Nutritional roles of lactoferrin. *Current Opinion in Clinical Nutrition & Metabolic Care*, *12*(3), 293-297.

39. Majka, G., Więcek, G., Śróttek, M., Śpiewak, K., Brindell, M., Koziel, J., & Strus, M. (2016). The impact of lactoferrin with different levels of metal saturation on the intestinal epithelial barrier function and mucosal inflammation. *BioMetals*, *29*(6), 1019-1033.

40. Moayyedi, P., & Cranney, A. (2008). Hip fracture and proton pump inhibitor therapy: balancing the evidence for benefit and harm. *The American journal of gastroenterology*, *103*(10), 2428-2431.

41. Norman, E. J. (1987). New urinary methylmalonic acid test is a sensitive indicator of cobalamin (vitamin B12) deficiency: a solution for a major unrecognized medical problem. *J Lab Clin Med*, *110*(369), b9.

42. Norman, E. J., Martelo, O. J., & Denton, M. D. (1982). Cobalamin (vitamin B12) deficiency detection by urinary methylmalonic acid quantitation. *Blood*, *59*(6), 1128-1131.

43. Parikh, S. J., Edelman, M., Uwaifo, G. I., Freedman, R. J., Semega-Janneh, M., Reynolds, J., & Yanovski, J. A. (2004). The relationship between obesity and serum 1, 25-dihydroxy vitamin D concentrations in healthy adults. *The Journal of Clinical Endocrinology & Metabolism*, *89*(3), 1196-1199.

44. Pierrot-Deseilligny, C., & Souberbielle, J. C. (2010). Is hypovitaminosis D one of the environmental risk factors for multiple sclerosis? *Brain*, *133*(7), 1869-1888.

45. Polotsky, H. N., & Polotsky, A. J. (2010, September). Metabolic implications of menopause. In *Seminars in reproductive medicine* (Vol. 28, No. 05, pp. 426-434). © Thieme Medical Publishers.

46. Raman, M., Milestone, A. N., Walters, J. R., Hart, A. L., & Ghosh, S. (2011). Vitamin D and gastrointestinal diseases: inflammatory bowel disease and colorectal cancer. *Therapeutic advances in gastroenterology*, *4*(1), 49-62.

47. Reynolds, E. (2006). Vitamin B12, folic acid, and the nervous system. *The lancet neurology*, *5*(11), 949-960.

48. Reynolds, E. H. (2002). Folic acid, ageing, depression, and dementia. *British Medical Journal*, *324*(7352), 1512.

49. Sampson, H. A., Mendelson, L., & Rosen, J. P. (1992). Fatal and near-fatal anaphylactic reactions to food in children and adolescents. *New England Journal of Medicine*, *327*(6), 380-384.

50. Shapses, S. A., & Sukumar, D. (2011). Protein intake during weight loss: effects on bone. In *Nutritional Influences on Bone Health* (pp. 27-33). Springer London.

51. Souberbielle, J. C., Body, J. J., Lappe, J. M., Plebani, M., Shoenfeld, Y., Wang, T. J., & Gandini, S. (2010). Vitamin D and

musculoskeletal health, cardiovascular disease, autoimmunity and cancer: recommendations for clinical practice. *Autoimmunity reviews, 9*(11), 709-715.

52. Szymczak, J., Bohdanowicz-Pawlak, A., Waszczuk, E., & Jakubowska, J. (2012). Low bone mineral density in adult patients with coeliac disease, Department of Endocrinology, Diabetology and Isotope Treatment, Wroclaw Medical University, Poland. *Polish Journal of Endocrinology, Tom/Volume 63*(4), 270-269.

53. Thompson, T. (2000). Folate, iron, and dietary fiber contents of the gluten-free diet. *Journal of the American Dietetic Association, 100*(11), 1389-1396.

54. Tikkakoski, S., Savilahti, E., & Kolho, K. L. (2007). Undiagnosed coeliac disease and nutritional deficiencies in adults screened in primary health care. *Scandinavian journal of gastroenterology, 42*(1), 60-65.

55. Van der Kraan, M. I., van Marle, J., Nazmi, K., Groenink, J., van't Hof, W., Veerman, E. C., & Amerongen, A. V. N. (2005). Ultra structural effects of antimicrobial peptides from bovine lactoferrin on the membranes of Candida albicans and Escherichia coli. *Peptides, 26*(9), 1537-1542.

56. Via, M. (2012). The malnutrition of obesity: micronutrient deficiencies that promote diabetes. *ISRN endocrinology, 2012.*

57. Xanthakos, S. A. (2009). Nutritional deficiencies in obesity and after bariatric surgery. *Pediatric Clinics of North America, 56*(5), 1105-1121.

58. Yang, Y. X., Lewis, J. D., Epstein, S., & Metz, D. C. (2006). Long-term proton pump inhibitor therapy and risk of hip fracture. *Jama, 296*(24), 2947-2953.

Cellular Respiration and Weight Gain Connection

1. Archer, S. L. (2013). Mitochondrial dynamics—mitochondrial fission and fusion in human diseases. *New England Journal of Medicine, 369*(23), 2236-2251.

2. Harper, M. E., & Seifert, E. L. (2008). Thyroid hormone effects on

mitochondrial energetics. *Thyroid, 18*(2), 145-156.

3. Harper, M. E., Dent, R., Monemdjou, S., Bézaire, V., Van Wyck, L., Wells, G., & McPherson, R. (2002). Decreased mitochondrial proton leak and reduced expression of uncoupling protein 3 in skeletal muscle of obese diet-resistant women. *Diabetes, 51*(8), 2459-2466.

4. Jones, D. S. (2005). *Textbook of functional medicine.* Institute for Functional Medicine. 30(1), 501-542

5. Kim, B. (2008). Thyroid hormone as a determinant of energy expenditure and the basal metabolic rate. *Thyroid, 18*(2), 141-144.

6. Kvetny, J., Bomholt, T., Pedersen, P., Wilms, L., Anthonsen, S., & Larsen, J. (2009). Thyroid hormone effect on human mitochondria measured by flow cytometry. *Scandinavian journal of clinical and laboratory investigation, 69*(7), 772-776.

7. Lowell, B. B., & Spiegelman, B. M. (2000). Towards a molecular understanding of adaptive thermogenesis. *Nature, 404*(6778), 652-660.

8. Morava, E., Rodenburg, R., van Essen, H. Z., Vries, M., & Smeitink, J. (2006). Dietary intervention and oxidative phosphorylation capacity. *Journal of inherited metabolic disease, 29*(4), 589-589.

9. Parikh, S., Saneto, R., Falk, M. J., Anselm, I., Cohen, B. H., & Haas, R. (2009). A modern approach to the treatment of mitochondrial disease. *Current treatment options in neurology, 11*(6), and 414.

10. Petersen, K. F., Befroy, D., Dufour, S., Dziura, J., Ariyan, C., Rothman, D. L., & Shulman, G. I. (2003). Mitochondrial dysfunction in the elderly: possible role in insulin resistance. *Science, 300*(5622), 1140-1142.

11. Short, K. R., Bigelow, M. L., Kahl, J., Singh, R., Coenen-Schimke, J., Raghavakaimal, S., & Nair, K. S. (2005). Decline in skeletal muscle mitochondrial function with aging in humans. *Proceedings of the National Academy of Sciences of the United States of America, 102*(15), 5618-5623.

12. Wortmann, S. B., Zweers-van Essen, H., Rodenburg, R. J., Van Den Heuvel, L. P., De Vries, M. C., Rasmussen-Conrad, E., ... & Morava, E. (2009). Mitochondrial energy production correlates with the age-related BMI. *Pediatric research, 65*(1), 103-108.

The Gut - Weight Gain connection

1. Amy Maxmen, (2012), Antibiotics Linked to Weight Gain; Changes in the gut microbiome from low-dose antibiotics caused mice to gain weight. Similar alterations in humans taking antibiotics, especially children, might be adding to the obesity epidemic.

2. Angelakis, E., Armougom, F., Million, M., & Raoult, D. (2012). The relationship between gut microbiota and weight gain in humans. *Future microbiology*, *7*(1), 91-109.

3. Armougom, F., Henry, M., Vialettes, B., Raccah, D., & Raoult, D. (2009). Monitoring bacterial community of human gut microbiota reveals an increase in Lactobacillus in obese patients and Methanogens in anorexic patients. *PloS one*, *4*(9), e7125.

4. Bäckhed, F., Fraser, C. M., Ringel, Y., Sanders, M. E., Sartor, R. B., Sherman, P. M., & Finlay, B. B. (2012). Defining a healthy human gut micro biome: current concepts, future directions, and clinical applications. *Cell host & microbe*, *12*(5), 611-622.

5. Bengmark, S. (2013). Nutrition of the critically ill—a 21st-century perspective. *Nutrients*, *5*(1), 162-207.

6. Blaser, M. J. (2014). Missing microbes. *New York: Henry Holt and Co.*

7. Fasano, A. (2011). Zonulin and its regulation of intestinal barrier function: the biological door to inflammation, autoimmunity, and cancer. *Physiological reviews*, *91*(1), 151-175.

8. Fasano, A. (2012). Leaky gut and autoimmune diseases. *Clinical reviews in allergy & immunology*, *42*(1), 71-78.

9. Fasano, A. (2012). Zonulin, regulation of tight junctions, and autoimmune diseases. *Annals of the New York Academy of Sciences*, *1258*(1), 25-33.

10. Hoffmann, C., Dollive, S., Grunberg, S., Chen, J., Li, H., Wu, G. D., & Bushman, F. D. (2013). Archaea and fungi of the human gut micro biome: correlations with diet and bacterial residents. *PloS one*, *8*(6), e66019.

11. Iliev, I. D., Funari, V. A., Taylor, K. D., Nguyen, Q., Reyes, C.

N., Strom, S. P., ... & Rotter, J. I. (2012). Interactions between commensal fungi and the C-type lectin receptor Dectin-1 influence colitis. *Science, 336*(6086), 1314-1317.

12. Ivanov, I. I., & Honda, K. (2012). Intestinal commensal microbes as immune modulators. *Cell host & microbe, 12*(4), 496-508.

13. Layden, B. T., Angueira, A. R., Brodsky, M., Durai, V., & Lowe, W. L. (2013). Short chain fatty acids and their receptors: new metabolic targets. *Translational Research, 161*(3), 131-140.

14. LeBlanc, J. G., Milani, C., de Giori, G. S., Sesma, F., Van Sinderen, D., & Ventura, M. (2013). Bacteria as vitamin suppliers to their host: a gut microbiota perspective. *Current opinion in biotechnology, 24*(2), 160-168.

15. Madara, J. L., & Trier, J. S. (1980). Structural abnormalities of jejunal epithelial cell membranes in celiac sprue. *Laboratory investigation, 43*(3), 254-261.

16. Million, M., Angelakis, E., Paul, M., Armougom, F., Leibovici, L., & Raoult, D. (2012). Comparative meta-analysis of the effect of Lactobacillus species on weight gain in humans and animals. *Microbial pathogenesis, 53*(2), 100-108.

17. Million, M., Maraninchi, M., Henry, M., Armougom, F., Richet, H., Carrieri, P., & Raoult, D. (2011). Obesity-associated gut microbiota is enriched in Lactobacillus reuteri and depleted in Bifidobacterium animalis and Methanobrevibacter smithii. *International journal of obesity, 36*(6), 817-825.

18. Molinaro, F., Paschetta, E., Cassader, M., Gambino, R., & Musso, G. (2012). Probiotics, prebiotics, energy balance, and obesity: mechanistic insights and therapeutic implications. *Gastroenterology Clinics of North America, 41*(4), 843-854.

19. Moreno-Navarrete, J. M., Sabater, M., Ortega, F., Ricart, W., & Fernandez-Real, J. M. (2012). Circulating zonulin, a marker of intestinal permeability, is increased in association with obesity-associated insulin resistance. *PloS one, 7*(5), e37160.

20. Mullin, G. E. (2015). *The Gut Balance Revolution: Boost Your Metabolism, Restore Your Inner Ecology, and Lose the Weight for Good!* Rodale.

21. Nadal, I., Santacruz, A., Marcos, A., Warnberg, J., Garagorri, M., Moreno, L. A., & Delgado, M. (2009). Shifts in clostridia, bacteroides and immunoglobulin-coating fecal bacteria associated with weight loss in obese adolescents. *International Journal of Obesity*, *33*(7), 758-767.

22. Ott, S. J., Kühbacher, T., Musfeldt, M., Rosenstiel, P., Hellmig, S., Rehman, A., & Schreiber, S. (2008). Fungi and inflammatory bowel diseases: alterations of composition and diversity. *Scandinavian journal of gastroenterology*, *43*(7), 831-841.

23. Plenge, R. M. (2010). Unlocking the pathogenesis of celiac disease: a genome-wide association study reports more than a dozen new susceptibility loci for celiac disease. Analysis of eQTL data from these and previously established risk loci sheds light on the genetic pathways underlying this common autoimmune disease. *Nature genetics*, *42*(4), 281-283.

24. Rodríguez, M. M., Pérez, D., Chaves, F. J., Esteve, E., Marin-Garcia, P., Xifra, G., & Portero-Otin, M. (2015). Obesity changes the human gut mycobiome. *Scientific reports*, *5*.

25. Schwiertz, A., Taras, D., Schäfer, K., Beijer, S., Bos, N. A., Donus, C., & Hardt, P. D. (2010). Microbiota and SCFA in lean and overweight healthy subjects. *Obesity*, *18*(1), 190-195.

26. Tilg, H., & Kaser, A. (2011). Gut microbiome, obesity, and metabolic dysfunction. *The Journal of clinical investigation*, *121*(6), 2126-2132.

27. Tremaroli, V., & Bäckhed, F. (2012). Functional interactions between the gut microbiota and host metabolism. *Nature*, *489*(7415), 242-249.

28. Wu, G. D., & Lewis, J. D. (2013). Analysis of the human gut microbiome and association with disease. *Clinical gastroenterology and hepatology: the official clinical practice journal of the American Gastroenterological Association*, *11*(7).

29. Zhang, H., DiBaise, J. K., Zuccolo, A., Kudrna, D., Braidotti, M., Yu, Y., & Krajmalnik-Brown, R. (2009). Human gut microbiota in obesity and after gastric bypass. *Proceedings of the National Academy of Sciences*, *106*(7), 2365-2370.

30. Zuo, H. J., Xie, Z. M., Zhang, W. W., Li, Y. R., Wang, W., Ding, X. B., & Pei, X. F. (2011). Gut bacteria alteration in obese people and its relationship with gene polymorphism. *World J Gastroenterol*, *17*(8), 1076-1081.

Sleep

1. Boston, C. P., Henderson, L., & Zimbardo, P. (1998). ANXIETY DISORDERS ASSOCIATION OF AMERICA.

2. Girardeau, G., Benchenane, K., Wiener, S. I., Buzsáki, G., & Zugaro, M. B. (2009). Selective suppression of hippocampal ripples impairs spatial memory. *Nature neuroscience*, *12*(10), 1222-1223.

3. Is Your Sleep Schedule Making You Fat? (2012). *Women's Health*. Retrieved 5 February 2017, from http://www.womenshealthmag. com/weight-loss/stop-weight-gain

4. Khosro, S., Alireza, S., Omid, A., & Forough, S. (2011). Night work and inflammatory markers. *Indian journal of occupational and environmental medicine*, *15*(1), 38. No 7

5. Kondracki, N. L. (2012). The Link between Sleep and Weight Gain. *Today's Dietitian*, *14*(6), 48-54.

6. Kumari, M., Badrick, E., Ferrie, J., Perski, A., Marmot, M., & Chandola, T. (2007). Self-reported sleep duration and sleep disturbance are independently associated with cortisol secretion in the Whitehall II study. *The Journal of Clinical Endocrinology & Metabolism*, *94*(12), 4801-4809.

7. Lavie, P., Kremerman, S., & Wiel, M. (1982). Sleep disorders and safety at work in industry workers. *Accident Analysis & Prevention*, *14*(4), 311-314.

8. Luboshitzky, R., Aviv, A., Hefetz, A., Herer, P., Shen-Orr, Z., Lavie, L., & Lavie, P. (2002). Decreased pituitary-gonadal secretion in men with obstructive sleep apnea. *The Journal of Clinical Endocrinology & Metabolism*, *87*(7), 3394-3398.

9. Malmberg, B., Kecklund, G., Karlson, B., Persson, R., Flisberg, P., & Ørbaek, P. (2010). Sleep and recovery in physicians on night call: a longitudinal field study. *BMC health services research*, *10*(1), 239.

10. National Heart, Lung, and Blood Institute, & National Institutes of Health. (2005). Your Guide to Healthy Sleep (NIH Publication No. 06-5271).

11. National Highway Traffic Safety Administration. (2015). Research on drowsy driving. *Accessed October, 20.*

12. Palma, J. A., Urrestarazu, E., & Iriarte, J. (2013). Sleep loss as risk factor for neurologic disorders: a review. *Sleep Medicine, 14*(3), 229-236.

13. Pandi-Perumal S.R, Gehrman P., Monti, J. M., & Monjan, A. A. (Eds.). (2009). *Principles and practice of geriatric sleep medicine.* University of Pennsylvania, Philadelphia.

14. Ruggiero, J. S., & Redeker, N. S. (2014). Effects of napping on sleepiness and sleep-related performance deficits in night-shift workers: a systematic review. *Biological research for nursing, 16*(2), 134-142.

15. Siebern, A. T., & Manber, R. (2010). Insomnia and its effective non-pharmacologic treatment. *Medical Clinics of North America, 94*(3), 581-591.

16. Sleep, Performance, and Public Safety. Healthy Sleep (2007). *U.S Department of Health and Human Services. Harvard Medical School.* Retrieved 5 February 2017, from http://healthysleep.med. harvard.edu/healthy/matters/consequences/sleep-performance-and-public-safety

The Hormones Connection

1. Bauman, E., & Friedlander, J. (2016). Eating for Health: a new system, not another diet—I. *NAMAH-The Journal of Integral Health.* Bauman College *23*(4).

2. Collins, J. J. (2006). Phytotherapeutic management of endocrine dysfunctions. *Nutrinews, 8*(1), 1-8.

3. Hyman, M. (2007). Systems biology, toxins, obesity, and functional medicine. *Alternative therapies in health and medicine, 13*(2), S134.

4. Lu, C., Toepel, K., Irish, R., Fenske, R. A., Barr, D. B., & Bravo, R.

(2006). Organic diets significantly lower children's dietary exposure to organophosphorus pesticides. *Environmental health perspectives*, 260-263.

5. Smith-Spangler, C., Brandeau, M. L., Hunter, G. E., Bavinger, J. C., Pearson, M., Eschbach, P. J., & Olkin, I. (2012). Are organic foods safer or healthier than conventional alternatives? A systematic review. *Annals of internal medicine*, *157*(5), 348-366.

6. http://www.rushcopley.com/app/files/public/2162/pdf-rcmg-environment-amd-hormones-presentation.pdf

7. https://www.asrm.org/uploadedFiles/ASRM_Content/News_and_Publications/Joint_Statements/Exposure%20to%20toxic%20environmental%20agents2013members(1).pdf

8. http://drhyman.com/downloads/Toxins-and-Obesity.pdf

The Adrenal-Cortisol-DHEA Connection

1. Andrews, R. C., Herlihy, O., Livingstone, D. E., Andrew, R., & Walker, B. R. (2002). Abnormal cortisol metabolism and tissue sensitivity to cortisol in patients with glucose intolerance. *The Journal of Clinical Endocrinology & Metabolism*, *87*(12), 5587-5593.

2. Baker, S. M., Bennett, P., Bland, J. S., Galland, L., Hedaya, R. J., Houston, M., & Vasquez, A. (2010). Textbook of Functional Medicine. *Gig Harbor, WA: The Institute for Functional Medicine*.

3. Epel, E. S., McEwen, B., Seeman, T., Matthews, K., Castellazzo, G., Brownell, K. D., & Ickovics, J. R. (2000). Stress and body shape: stress-induced cortisol secretion is consistently greater among women with central fat. *Psychosomatic medicine*, *62*(5), 623-632.

4. Epel, E., Lapidus, R., McEwen, B., & Brownell, K. (2001). Stress may add bite to appetite in women: a laboratory study of stress-induced cortisol and eating behavior. *Psychoneuroendocrinology*, *26*(1), 37-49.

5. Westerbacka, J., Yki-Järvinen, H., Vehkavaara, S., Häkkinen, A. M., Andrew, R., Wake, D. J., & Walker, B. R. (2003). Body fat distribution and cortisol metabolism in healthy men: enhanced 5β-reductase and lower cortisol/cortisone metabolite ratios in

men with fatty liver. *The Journal of Clinical Endocrinology & Metabolism, 88*(10), 4924-4931.

Insulin Resistance

1. Acheson, K. J., Schutz, Y., Bessard, T., Anantharaman, K. R. I. S. H. N. A., Flatt, J. P., & Jequier, E. (1988). Glycogen storage capacity and de novo lipogenesis during massive carbohydrate overfeeding in man. *The American journal of clinical nutrition, 48*(2), 240-247.

2. Kahn, S. E., Hull, R. L., & Utzschneider, K. M. (2006). Mechanisms linking obesity to insulin resistance and type 2 diabetes. *Nature, 444*(7121), 840-846.

3. Mcfarlane, S. I., Banerji, M., & Sowers, J. R. (2001). Insulin Resistance and Cardiovascular Disease 1. *The Journal of Clinical Endocrinology & Metabolism, 86*(2), 713-718.

4. Nelson, D. L., Lehninger, A. L., & Cox, M. M. (2008). *Lehninger principles of biochemistry*. Macmillan.

5. Stanhope, K. L., Schwarz, J. M., Keim, N. L., Griffen, S. C., Bremer, A. A., Graham, J. L., ... & McGahan, J. P. (2009). Consuming fructose-sweetened, not glucose-sweetened, beverages increases visceral adiposity and lipids and decreases insulin sensitivity in overweight/obese humans. *The Journal of clinical investigation, 119*(5), 1322-1334.

Sex Hormone Connections

1. Bhasin S, et al. (2007). *J Clin Endocrinol Metab. 92(3):1049-57*

2. Boyanov MA, et al., (2003). Aging Male. *6(1):1-7.*

3. Chen RY, et al., (2006). *Diabetes Obes Metab. 8(4):429-35*

4. Cohen PG, (2008). Med Hypotheses. *70(2):358-60.*

5. Dandona P, et al., (2008). *Curr Mol Med. 8(8):816-28.*

6. Diaz-Arjonilla M, (2009). *Int J Impot Res Mar 21(2):89-98.*

7. Haider A, et al., (2009). Andrologia. *41(1):7-13*

8. Kaplan SA, et al., (2006). *Journal of Urol. 176(4 Pt. 1):1524-7;* discussion *27-8*

9. Laaksonen DE, et al., (2004). Diabetes Care. *27(5):1036-41*

10. Lunenfeld B. (2007). Aging Male. *10(2):53-6.*

11. Lunenfeld B., (2007). Testosterone deficiency and the metabolic syndrome, Aging Male, 10(2):53-6

12. Makhsida N, et al., (2005*). J Urol. 174(3):827-34.*

13. Muller M, et al., (2005). *J Clin Endocrinol Metab. 90(5):2618-23*

14. Nelson LR, et al., (2001). *Journal of America Academy Derm 45(3): 116-24.*

15. Niskanen, L., Laaksonen, D. E., Punnonen, K., Mustajoki, P., Kaukua, J., & Rissanen, A. (2004). Changes in sex hormone-binding globulin and testosterone during weight loss and weight maintenance in abdominally obese men with the metabolic syndrome. *Diabetes, Obesity and Metabolism, 6*(3), 208-215.

16. Rind, B., (2009). *Estrogen Dominance.* Retrieved from: http://www.drrind.com/therapies/estrogen-dominance

17. Spark RF, (2007). *Curr Urol Rep. 8(6):467-71.*

18. Traish AM, et al., (2009). *J Androl. 30(1):23-32*

19. *Zumoff B. Acta Med Scand Suppl. 1988; 723:153-60.*

Thyroid Connection

1. Canaris, G. J., Manowitz, N. R., Mayor, G., & Ridgway, E. C. (2000). The Colorado thyroid disease prevalence study. *Archives of internal medicine, 160*(4), 526-534.

2. Feart, C., Pallet, V., Boucheron, C., Higueret, D., Alfos, S., Letenneur, L., & Higueret, P. (2005). Aging affects the retinoic acid and the triiodothyronine nuclear receptor mRNA expression in human peripheral blood mononuclear cells. *European Journal of Endocrinology, 152*(3), 449-458.

3. Nishiyama, S., Inomoto, T., Nakamura, T., Higashi, A., & Matsuda, I. (1996). Zinc status relates to hematological deficits in women endurance runners. *Journal of the American College of Nutrition*, *15*(4), 359-363.

4. Olivieri O, Girelli D, et al., (1996). Biological Trace Element Research, 51:31--41

5. Roti, E., Minelli, R., & Salvi, M. (2000). Thyroid hormone metabolism in obesity. *International journal of obesity*, *24*, S113-S115.

6. Wartofsky, L., Van Nostrand, D., & Burman, K. D. (2006). Overt and 'subclinical' hypothyroidism in women. *Obstetrical & gynecological survey*, *61*(8), 535-542.

Leptin and Ghrelin References

1. Brennan, A. M., & Mantzoros, C. S. (2006). Drug Insight: the role of leptin in human physiology and pathophysiology—emerging clinical applications. *Nature Reviews Endocrinology*, *2*(6), 318-327.

2. Considine, R. V., Sinha, M. K., Heiman, M. L., Kriauciunas, A., Stephens, T. W., Nyce, M. R., & Caro, J. F. (1996). Serum immunoreactive-leptin concentrations in normal-weight and obese humans. *New England Journal of Medicine*, *334*(5), 292-295.

3. Copinschi G1, Leproult *R, Spiegel K., (2014)*. The importantrole of sleep in metabolism, Front Hormone Research, 42:59-72

4. Folgueira C1, Seoane LM, Casanueva FF, (2014). Front Hormone Research, 42:83-92

5. Lustig, R. H., Sen, S., Soberman, J. E., & Velasquez-Mieyer, P. A. (2004). Obesity, leptin resistance, and the effects of insulin reduction. *International journal of obesity*, *28*(10), 1344-1348.

6. Murray, S., Tulloch, A., Gold, M. S., & Avena, N. M. (2014). Hormonal and neural mechanisms of food reward, eating behaviour and obesity. *Nature Reviews Endocrinology*, *10*(9), 540-552.

7. Weigle, D. S., Cummings, D. E., Newby, P. D., Breen, P. A., Frayo, R. S., Matthys, C. C., ... & Purnell, J. Q. (2003). Roles of

leptin and ghrelin in the loss of body weight caused by a low fat, high carbohydrate diet. *The Journal of Clinical Endocrinology & Metabolism, 88*(4), 1577-1586.

Balanced Diet

1. Acheson, K. J., Zahorska-Markiewicz, B., Pittet, P., Anantharaman, K., & Jéquier, E. (1980). Caffeine and coffee: their influence on metabolic rate and substrate utilization in normal weight and obese individuals. *The American journal of clinical nutrition, 33*(5), 989-997.

2. Afify, A. E. M. M., El-Beltagi, H. S., El-Salam, S. M. A., & Omran, A. A. (2011). Bioavailability of iron, zinc, phytate and phytase activity during soaking and germination of white sorghum varieties. *Plos one, 6*(10), e25512.

3. Altieri, A., La Vecchia, C., & Negri, E. (2003). Fluid intake and risk of bladder and other cancers. *European journal of clinical nutrition, 57*, S59-S68.

4. Baillie, R. A., Takada, R., Nakamura, M., & Clarke, S. D. (1999). Coordinate induction of peroxisomal acyl-CoA oxidase and UCP-3 by dietary fish oil: a mechanism for decreased body fat deposition. *Prostaglandins, leukotrienes and essential fatty acids, 60*(5-6), 351-356.

5. Belzung, F., Raclot, T., & Groscolas, R. (1993). Fish oil n-3 fatty acids selectively limit the hypertrophy of abdominal fat depots in growing rats fed high-fat diets. *American Journal of Physiology-Regulatory, Integrative and Comparative Physiology, 264*(6), R1111-R1118.

6. Blatt, A. D., Roe, L. S., & Rolls, B. J. (2011). Increasing the protein content of meals and its effect on daily energy intake. *Journal of the American Dietetic Association, 111*(2), 290-294.

7. Buckley, J. D., & Howe, P. R. (2010). Long-chain omega-3 polyunsaturated fatty acids may be beneficial for reducing obesity—a review. *Nutrients, 2*(12), 1212-1230.

8. Cameron, E. A., Kwiatkowski, K. J., Lee, B. H., Hamaker, B. R., Koropatkin, N. M., & Martens, E. C. (2014). Multifunctional

nutrient-binding proteins adapt human symbiotic bacteria for glycan competition in the gut by separately promoting enhanced sensing and catalysis. *MBio*, *5*(5), e01441-14.

9. Conlon, M. A., & Bird, A. R. (2015). The impact of diet and lifestyle on gut micro biota and human health. *Nutrients*, *7*(1), 17-44.

10. Cunnane, S. C., McAdoo, K. R., & Horrobin, D. F. (1986). N-3 Essential fatty acids decrease weight gain in genetically obese mice. *British journal of nutrition*, *56*(01), 87-95.

11. Cutler, E., Ellen W. & Kaslow E. (2005). *Micro Miracles: Discover the Healing Power of Enzymes*. Rodale.

12. Flint, H. J., Scott, K. P., Duncan, S. H., Louis, P., & Forano, E. (2012). Microbial degradation of complex carbohydrates in the gut. *Gut microbes*, *3*(4), 289-306.

13. Grandjean, A.C., & Grandjean N.R. (2007). Dehydration and cognitive performance. *Journal of the American College of Nutrition*, Vol. 26, 549-554.

14. Gupta, R. K., Gangoliya, S. S., & Singh, N. K. (2015). Reduction of phytic acid and enhancement of bioavailable micronutrients in food grains. *Journal of food science and technology*, *52*(2), 676-684.

15. Hainault, I., Carlotti, M., Hajduch, E., Guichard, C., & Lavau, M. (1993). Fish oil in a high lard diet prevents obesity, hyperlipemia, and adipocyte insulin resistance in rats. *Annals of the New York Academy of Sciences*, *683*(1), 98-101.

16. Hughes, J., & Norman, R. W. (1992). Diet and calcium stones. *CMAJ: Canadian Medical Association Journal*, *146*(2), 137.

17. Johnston, C. S., Day, C. S., & Swan, P. D. (2002). Postprandial thermogenesis is increased 100% on a high-protein, low-fat diet versus a high-carbohydrate, low-fat diet in healthy, young women. *Journal of the American College of Nutrition*, *21*(1), 55-61.

18. Kalsbeek, A., la Fleur, S., & Fliers, E. (2014). Circadian control of glucose metabolism. *Molecular metabolism*, *3*(4), 372-383.

19. Kanerva, N., Kaartinen, N. E., Schwab, U., Lahti-Koski, M., & Männistö, S. (2013). Adherence to the Baltic Sea diet consumed in

the Nordic countries is associated with lower abdominal obesity. *British Journal of Nutrition, 109*(03), 520-528.

20. Lane, J. D. (2011). Caffeine, glucose metabolism, and type 2 diabetes. *Journal of Caffeine Research, 1*(1), 23-28.

21. Lieber, C. S. (1989). Alcohol and nutrition; an overview. *Alcohol Health & Research World, 13*(3), 197-206.

22. Lovallo, W. R., Whitsett, T. L., al'Absi, M., Sung, B. H., Vincent, A. S., & Wilson, M. F. (2011) Stimulation of Cortisol Secretion Across the Waking Hours in Relation to Caffeine Intake Levels; *Journal of Caffeine Research,* 1(1): 23-28.

23. Macfarlane, G. T., & Macfarlane, S. (2012). Bacteria, colonic fermentation, and gastrointestinal health. *Journal of AOAC International, 95*(1), 50-60.

24. Marmonier, C., Chapelot, D., Fantino, M., & Louis-Sylvestre, J. (2002). Snacks consumed in a nonhungry state have poor satiating efficiency: influence of snack composition on substrate utilization and hunger. *The American journal of clinical nutrition, 76*(3), 518-528.

25. Montani, J. P., Viecelli, A. K., Prévot, A., & Dulloo, A. G. (2006). Weight cycling during growth and beyond as a risk factor for later cardiovascular diseases: the 'repeated overshoot 'theory. *International Journal of Obesity, 30*, S58-S66.

26. Mozaffarian, D., Katan, M. B., Ascherio, A., Stampfer, M. J., & Willett, W. C. (2006). Trans-fatty acids and cardiovascular disease. *New England Journal of Medicine, 354*(15), 1601-1613.

27. Osterweil, N., & Mathis, C. E. G. (2004). The Benefits of Protein. Retrieved June 1, 2010, from http://www.webmd.com/fitness-exercise/guide/benefitsprotein

28. Peek, C. B., Ramsey, K. M., Marcheva, B., & Bass, J. (2012). Nutrient sensing and the circadian clock. *Trends in Endocrinology & Metabolism, 23*(7), 312-318.

29. Ruzickova, J., Rossmeisl, M., Prazak, T., Flachs, P., Sponarova, J., Vecka, M., & Kopecky, J. (2004). Omega-3 PUFA of marine origin limits diet-induced obesity in mice by reducing cellularity of

adipose tissue. *Lipids, 39*(12), 1177-1185.

30. Sacks, F. M., Bray, G. A., Carey, V. J., Smith, S. R., Ryan, D. H., Anton, S. D., ... & Leboff, M. S. (2009). Comparison of weight-loss diets with different compositions of fat, protein, and carbohydrates. *N Engl J Med, 2009*(360), 859-873.

31. Shimizu, M., Payne, C. R., & Wansink, B. (2010). When snacks become meals: How hunger and environmental cues bias food intake. *International Journal of Behavioral Nutrition and Physical Activity, 7*(1), 63.

32. Strohacker, K., & McFarlin, B. K. (2009). Influence of obesity, physical inactivity, and weight cycling on chronic inflammation. *Frontiers in bioscience (Elite edition), 2*, 98-104.

33. Tang, D., Dong, Y., Ren, H., Li, L., & He, C. (2014). A review of phytochemistry, metabolite changes, and medicinal uses of the common food mung bean and its sprouts (Vigna radiata). *Chemistry Central Journal, 8*(1), 4.

34. Valtin, H. (2002). "Drink at least eight glasses of water a day." Really? Is there scientific evidence for "8× 8"? *American Journal of Physiology-Regulatory, Integrative and Comparative Physiology, 283*(5), R993-R1004.

35. Veldhorst, M. A., Westerterp, K. R., van Vught, A. J., & Westerterp-Plantenga, M. S. (2010). Presence or absence of carbohydrates and the proportion of fat in a high-protein diet affect appetite suppression but not energy expenditure in normal-weight human subjects fed in energy balance. *British journal of nutrition, 104*(09), 1395-1405.

36. Weigle, D. S., Breen, P. A., Matthys, C. C., Callahan, H. S., Meeuws, K. E., Burden, V. R., & Purnell, J. Q. (2005). A high-protein diet induces sustained reductions in appetite, ad libitum caloric intake, and body weight despite compensatory changes in diurnal plasma leptin and ghrelin concentrations. *The American journal of clinical nutrition, 82*(1), 41-48.

37. Wells, H. F., & Buzby, J. C. (2008). Dietary assessment of major trends in US food consumption, *1970-2005*. Washington: *US Department of Agriculture, Economic Research Service.*

38. Wild, T., Rahbarnia, A., Kellner, M., Sobotka, L., & Eberlein, T.

(2009). Centers for Disease Control and Prevention. *Nutrition, 26*(9), 862-866.

39. Wycherley, T. P., Moran, L. J., Clifton, P. M., Noakes, M., & Brinkworth, G. D. (2012). Effects of energy-restricted high-protein, low-fat compared with standard-protein, low-fat diets: a meta-analysis of randomized controlled trials. *The American journal of clinical nutrition*, ajcn-044321.

40. Zieve, D. (2009, May 2). In Protein in diet: MedlinePlus Medical Encyclopedia. Retrieved June 1, 2010, from http://www.nlm.nih.gov/

41. http://online.liebertpub.com/doi/abs/10.1089/jcr.2010.0007

42. http://pubs.niaaa.nih.gov/publications/aa22.htm

Visit: www.mor-nutrition4life.com

89292154R00167

Made in the USA
Columbia, SC
12 February 2018